Praise for Excellence in the Emergency Department

"For those of us who have chosen a career in emergency care, Stephanie's insight, wisdom, and passion for patient care are an inspiration. If we truly believe that the ED is the front door to the hospital for our patients, her detailed explanation of why we should do better, how we can create change, and description of the methods to stay at the highest level of performance are crucial reading for all ED and hospital leaders."
—Jeff Wood, RN, Southwest Regional Director, EmCare

"Stephanie was my Studer coach when I was a hospital CEO...and I knew I had the 'cream of the crop.' She has taken her experience in the ED, a high level of emotional intelligence, and her own practical approach to driving results...and she has written this wonderful book. If the concepts and 'prescriptives' were followed, anyone could be proud of their own ED of Excellence that produces great results."
—Barbara Blevins, COO, Team Health

"*Excellence in the Emergency Department* provides a road map in the navigation and implementation of change leading to a high performing ED."
—Roger Brooksbank, MD, Regional Medical Director, Team Health

"*Excellence in the Emergency Department: How to Get Results* provides a practical approach to improving outcomes in all pillars of ED operations, including people, service, quality, finance, and growth. Stephanie Baker 'AIDETs' her way through a clear, concise message and a call to action for ED managers. I highly recommend this book for all ED managers, new or experienced. *Excellence in the Emergency Department: How to Get Results* outlines the strategies that Stephanie Baker used that helped us bring our ED from the 9th to the 99th percentile in patient satisfaction. Over a year later, we are still experiencing high levels of patient satisfaction, lower left without treatment rates, higher staff retention, and continued volume growth."
—Kris Powell, RN, ED Director, Baylor Regional Medical Center-Grapevine

"Stephanie understands the unique complexity and needs of the Emergency Department. Stephanie has written a book that will move your department from good to great. She will teach you how to set realistic goals and how to measure and achieve those goals. Stephanie has captured the essence of what all Emergency Departments that want to achieve and sustain excellence in patient satisfaction are all about."
—Diana Shaffer, RN, ED Manager, Parkwest Medical Center

"Managing an Emergency Department is tough. Often, it is more like a war zone than a hospital. Most people believe it can't have the high patient satisfaction scores the rest of the institution strives to achieve. This book challenges that notion. Stephanie Baker skillfully presents Studer Group's proven approach to performance improvement customized for this toughest of environments. The result is a book that's as reassuring as it is instructive. A great read for anyone responsible for ED operations."
—Greg Pivirotto, President and CEO, University Medical Center, Arizona

Excellence in the Emergency Department

How to Get Results

Stephanie J. Baker, RN, CEN, MBA

Published by:
Fire Starter Publishing
913 Gulf Breeze Parkway, Suite 6
Gulf Breeze, FL 32561
Phone: 850-934-1099
Fax: 850-934-1384
www.firestarterpublishing.com

ISBN: 978-0-9840794-8-3

Library of Congress Control Number: 2009934548

Printed in the United States of America

I dedicate this book to:

My parents, Saul and Sue, whose unconditional love for me prompted them to make life-altering choices that forever changed the course of my life and health for the better. Thank you for the sacrifices you made then and continue to make now for our family. I am undeniably blessed to have you as my parents. You two are my True North.

My sister, Angela, who consistently role-models what I want to be...kind, loving, generous, forgiving, compassionate, and, above all, uplifting to each person she comes in contact with. Had I been given the choice to personally select my one and only sister, I would have chosen you. Thankfully, God chose you for me!

Emergency caregivers everywhere. Your passion and commitment are second to none. The lives of our patients are better because of the work you do every day. Stay the course, promote the profession, and commit to leading the way.

Table of Contents

Reasons for resistance to change in the Emergency Department
Overcoming barriers and driving out negativity
Dealing with low performers

The quality/service connection
Evidence-Based Leadership℠
Financial impact

The Healthcare Flywheel®
The external market: Are you unique?
The five pillars: A balanced approach to getting results

Leader rounding on staff
Leader rounding on patients
Rounding in the ED waiting room/reception area

Why to make the calls
How to make the calls
Who makes the calls

Foreword

Emergency Departments are many times the front door or the entry point to healthcare today. People are not timid if they feel their ED visit was too long or they felt ignored or they didn't understand what they heard—they will share this with the community. As healthcare providers, we know when we are out in the community when people are pleased with the care they receive and when they are not.

In my healthcare experience, I have found that many times the community's impression of the hospital is generally based on the Emergency Department. The Emergency Department is a great place to create positive word of mouth and most importantly save lives.

To have a great ED, the rest of the organization has to be running well. Are there beds available? Are the test results there? So when we're talking about the ED, we're really not talking solely about the ED but the efficiency of the entire organization. There are specific things you can do in the ED, but of course it's only one part of the comprehensive picture. It's important to really manage patient flow from beginning to end as it applies to your entire organization. When I was a COO at Holy Cross in Chicago, it was my great opportunity to see an ED transformed in what many would consider a tough inner-city with a high self-pay client base. Once again, as president of Baptist Hospital, Inc., in Pensacola, FL, I watched an ED transform from less than 1 percentile in patient perception of care to a 99 percentile in patient perception of care. I also witnessed a tremendous reduction in people leaving without being treated, ability to collect co-pays, and an increase in volume. Our research has shown that when more patients choose your ED, your payor mix gets better because it is the payor who many times won't come if there is a reputation of high wait times or will leave for another alternative if it looks like it is taking too long.

When the ED is running well, the most important thing happens: Lives are saved with improved clinical quality by reducing staff and physician turnover.

So for years Studer Group® has focused in on EDs by having ED experts on staff who came from running successful Emergency Departments—from operating our Nuts and Bolts two-day institute on running the Emergency Department to having ED physicians on staff as medical directors. We've been in EDs from the smallest towns to the largest cities in the U.S. We've worked with EDs from Alaska to Miami; from Bangor, Maine, to San Diego. What we have found is that while each one is different, there are tools and tactics that work in every ED to improve performance.

When I was the keynote speaker at the Emergency Nurse Association's (ENA) National Conference, it was very apparent there was no shortage of passion and no shortage of will. There was also no shortage of desire to find out what tools, techniques, and skills are needed to have great Emergency Departments. I am thrilled that Stephanie Baker has taken the time and energy to share her own experiences and collect from our SG experts on staff, other experts in the industry, and hundreds of experts in EDs that we work with to put together a comprehensive toolkit that takes the complexity of running a great ED and simplifies it into key tactics that can be executed.

People who work in the Emergency Department have the ability to handle a range of emotions most could not. They deserve a great place to work. Patients who come to the Emergency Department deserve a great place to receive care. That is what this book is all about: making the Emergency Department a great place for employees to work and patients to receive care. Thank you for your dedication to making healthcare better.

—Quint Studer

Introduction

From the time I was a small child, I always wanted to be a nurse. But not just any nurse, an emergency nurse.

Perhaps it was the frequency with which I visited my doctor's office and the Emergency Department as a child. Born and raised until the age of nine in Lexington, Kentucky, I suffered from severe allergies and asthma that kept me in close contact with my pediatrician and gave me frequent opportunity to experience the healthcare system.

It's true that things were different in the late Sixties and early Seventies, but one thing that has stayed the same is the passion and commitment I felt from the nurses and physicians who treated me then and those who I coach today.

It was rough in those early years. As a child, you want to run and play, not take medicine and breathing treatments. My caregivers cared a great deal about me and my family and kept trying different courses of treatment that might help. I remember my dad pleading with my pediatrician to give me something to make me feel better. He said he would do anything to help me live a better life. The advice my doctor gave my dad that day changed our lives forever and would draw me closer to my career in emergency medicine.

Dr. Penn shared with my dad that Kentucky was not the ideal climate for someone with my medical condition and that moving to a drier, more temperate climate would likely improve my health. Since my mom had severe bronchitis (as well as osteoarthritis that she was diagnosed with at an early age), my parents began to look for a place to relocate our family.

After my mom wrote to the National Weather Service (as those were the days before the Internet) and reviewed their recommendations, all roads seemed to lead to either Tucson, Arizona, or San Diego, California. My dad eventually loaded everything we owned in a U-Haul truck, put my sister and me in the family station wagon with my mom, and we headed west. It was quite the adventure for a family who had never been west of the Mississippi, had limited financial resources, and no current promise of employment for either of my parents. What we did have was our strong Christian faith and hope for a healthier future.

As fate would have it, July was the month we made the trip. It was hot and uncomfortable and the weather didn't seem to improve as we traveled towards the west coast. When we stopped in Tucson, Arizona, it was 118 degrees in the shade!

I remember my dad pumping gas and the sweat just pouring down his face. He looked at my mom and said, "We can't stay here!" and our journey continued. When we finally arrived in San Diego, it felt like heaven. The weather was glorious. Within six months my allergies were gone, my asthma had greatly improved, and I was off all of my medication!

The years passed and life happened. I fulfilled my dream to become a nurse and graduated with my Bachelor of Science degree in Nursing from San Diego State University in 1988. I literally "begged" my way into my first job as an Emergency Department nurse.

Those were the days before the nursing shortage. I had to work hard to convince my manager that I could do the job. My orientation might be described as similar to a sorority "hazing" process, but somehow I survived and loved every minute of it!

The next 17 years were filled with days (and many nights) in Emergency Departments, trauma units, ground and air transport vehicles, and even jail detention facilities (but that's another story). My experience led me into leadership positions that offered the opportunity to effect change, improve quality of patient care, advocate for staff, partner with physicians, and build strong relationships with administration. I never felt I had a job. For me, it was always a calling.

In 2005, I attended an Emergency Department conference hosted by Studer Group, where I met Jay Kaplan, MD, and Julie Kennedy, RN. Those two days re-ignited my passion to make a difference in emergency medicine, and I was practically floating on air as I boarded my plane home thinking of all the things I had learned that could make our Emergency Department better.

In a lucky stroke of synchronicity, Jay happened to be on my plane as he had a speaking engagement in San Diego the following day. When he saw me, he asked the woman seated next to me if he could trade seats with her. He was interested in learning more about the work we had done to reduce wait times and improve our patient experience in our large inner-city ED.

Needless to say, the two hours flew by! After landing, Jay gave me his card and said, "We need someone like you." He encouraged me to submit my résumé for a coaching position with Studer Group. As a result, for the last four years, I have been a coach, account leader, and national speaker with Studer Group, working with healthcare organizations all across the country to improve operational and service efficiency, particularly in the ED. Jay, I am forever grateful to you for that plane ride!

I believe that most ED leaders want to pay it forward when it comes to the mentoring, experience, and assistance they have received. That is my hope for this book: to put the tools and tactics that I have seen work in so many EDs in your hands.

And I urge you: Don't waste a moment feeling badly for expecting excellence in your ED. Whether you're a leader, a physician, a staff nurse, or an ED technician, your team needs you to role-model it. You owe it to your patients.

Here's what I've learned: Sometimes we get only one chance. Over the past 20 years, I've cared for thousands of patients and there were so many times that I knew I'd be the last face that patient would see...the last person to help them die with dignity...the last person to help manage their pain…the last person to carry a message to their family or friends.

There are *no* bad days in emergency medicine. It has to be *every* patient *every* time. It's a sacred vocation that we're charged with… one of the most rewarding I've ever found.

In the following pages, I look forward to sharing with you evidence-based tools and tactics that will ignite your passion for what you do and create the kind of environment where employees want to work, physicians want to practice, and patients want to receive care. So be encouraged.

Excellence in the Emergency Department is within reach. Is it easy? No. Is it necessary? Yes. Great leaders do the hard stuff. Good leaders follow others. And poor leaders make excuses.

If you're reading this book, you already have the passion and the will to make the changes necessary to create excellence in your ED. You already know the "why." This book will give you the "how."

So be strong. Be committed. Be relentless. And as they said on 9/11, "Let's roll!"

Fantasy or Reality?

Imagine with me for a moment…

You—the patient—arrive at the ED and are immediately greeted by a professional triage nurse who quickly assesses your condition. After this brief interaction, you are escorted to a bed in the ED where a courteous member of the registration staff comes to your bedside to take your demographic information and provides you with a written copy of the hospital's privacy policies.

Within five minutes the ED physician comes in, introduces herself, gives you some brief information about her experience, and proceeds by asking pertinent questions about your chief complaint, followed by a physical exam.

The physician then describes what course of action is planned and lets you know what to expect, including how long you will likely stay in the ED. Within a few minutes, the nurse arrives to provide treatments and medication ordered by the physician. He introduces himself, explains what is going to take place, and offers to have your family member join you at the bedside while you wait for further tests. The nurse pays special attention to your personal needs and makes sure you are comfortable while you are waiting, promising to return at least once every hour to assess your pain and keep you updated on your plan of care and what to expect next.

As different staff members enter the room to perform treatments or take you for ordered tests, each person provides an introduction and explains what is going to happen and how long each procedure will take. As promised, the nurse or ED technician returns to the bedside hourly to assess your level of pain and provides an update on your plan of care and what you are waiting for.

Once all of the test results are available, the ED physician returns and sits at your bedside to explain the test results, diagnosis, and plan of care. The good news is that you will be able to go home! Once the physician has written the discharge orders, the nurse returns to provide thorough instructions and asks what questions you have. The nurse thanks you for choosing their organization and advises you that someone will be calling you in the next 72 hours to make sure you are doing well at home. The ED technician escorts you to your car and ends the interaction by asking, "Is there anything else I can do for you?"

Perhaps this ED experience sounds like a fantasy, especially in light of what is often shared in the newspaper and on television. The good news is that this type of experience is a reality in hundreds of EDs across America that are embracing Studer Group's "Must Have" behaviors to build a culture of excellence and accountability.

This book will provide you with the practical "how to's" for implementing the behaviors that are helping so many EDs to become the best place for employees to work, physicians to practice, and patients to receive care.

There is no magic wand to wave or fairy dust to sprinkle: just simple evidence-based tools and tactics that produce sustained results when used consistently. By purchasing this book, you have taken the first step to embark on this journey to excellence. As you turn the page, hold on tight. The best is yet to come!

"Why Change?"

CHAPTER 1

The Resistance Reality

"Resistance is thought transformed into feeling. Change the thought that creates the resistance, and there is no more resistance."
—Robert Conklin

In today's healthcare environment, change is the only constant. There are reimbursement changes. Regulatory changes. Economic changes. More patients than ever. But, as the external operating environment gets increasingly difficult, great leaders understand the need to adapt to survive and thrive in the future.

Ultimately, leaders are responsible for driving change. So it's important that we hold up the mirror and commit to it. Change begins with us...with how well we position change and role model it. It's important to explain to staff that we are embracing change to respond to the external operating environment and because the literature shows us that adopting new evidence-based practices will deliver better clinical and quality outcomes for patients. If, instead, leaders position change as something required by administration, they can create a "we/they" culture that will sink their efforts.

In fact, the sign of a true leader is his or her ability to develop a process for change, show others why they need to change, and execute change. Results come by working through processes, not being fearful of risk, and successfully engaging staff.

But sometimes we find that even if we, as leaders, are committed to change, our staff just won't fall in line. Why are they so resistant? And can we succeed in the face of such resistance? The answer is yes!

Having worked with staff and leaders in hundreds of Emergency Departments, at Studer Group® we know that ED folks are survivors. They have passion for what they do every day. And there are concrete reasons why they sometimes resist change.

Let's examine a few:

It's risky to change.[1] Changing behaviors is risky. But often, it's riskier to do nothing. At Studer Group, we frequently find that there is a large gap between the urgency that senior leaders feel to make changes that respond to the current economic and regulatory environment and the urgency felt by middle managers and staff. Because they don't understand that the pressures for change are external, staff frequently feel the pressure as an internal one that is coming from their supervisors. Instead of teaming up to respond to external factors that threaten the organization, people can end up resenting their leaders (more "we/they") and feel like they're just being asked to do one more thing.

The purpose for change is not clear. Similar to the above, we as leaders don't always communicate the "why" in a way that will engage our employees. Most of our staff want to do a good job and really care about their patients, but they may feel overwhelmed with too much to do already. Just as Studer Group recommends telling a patient why you are closing a curtain (e.g., "for your privacy"), it's also important to tell your employees how the new behaviors you are asking them to use connect to things they care about (e.g., patient safety, better clinical outcomes, a better workplace, more efficiency, more time).

They feel they lack the staff. With tight budgets, fewer nursing graduates, and many leaving the profession, ED staffing shortages are common. Perhaps you have a dedicated manager who just doesn't feel he has the critical mass in the department to get and sustain results. At Studer Group, we find that when ED leaders are transparent about their staffing models and share data with employees, they will engage and become part of the process to match staff to patient flow. Frequently, it is not a question of having enough staff, but how efficiently existing staff is being used.

There is fear of failure. Employees wonder, *Can I do it?* or *I don't know how* or *We already tried that, and it didn't work.* We are famous in the ED for identifying a problem on Friday ("We've just got to do something about that!") and implementing a solution on Monday. But the lack of planning, training, discipline, and follow-through can doom our execution, leaving staff disenchanted. A little training and planning will go a long way towards sustained success.

While we're not going to boil the ocean tomorrow, we *can* chip away at small steps of change for long-term dramatic results. (Don't be afraid to pilot-test a new process!) But to prevail, we will need the right people at the table...including your internal customers. (See Chapter 9: Interdepartmental Communication Tools.)

They lack the will. While most of your employees are passionate about their work, you probably also have some low performers. Low performers tend to be especially resistant to change because change means more effort and they might lose their power base.

Ask yourself: *Is it a question of skill or will?* If your staff lack skill, then are they teachable? If so, training is the answer. If it's a lack of will, do they understand the why and do they have the passion to overcome this barrier? You'll need to connect to purpose, set clear expectations, and hold low-performing employees accountable with an "up or out" approach.

Why People Don't Do What We Want Them To[2]

Don't know **what** to do
(knowledge expectations)

Don't know **how** to do it
(ability/skill)

Don't know **why** they should do it
(importance)

Don't **want** to
(lack of will)

Aren't **well-suited** or matched to the task
(selection)

Overcoming Barriers and Driving Out Negativity

Once you understand the reasons for resistance, you can address them. In fact, the main ways to effectively address employee resistance are: 1) strong communication, 2) effective training, and 3) consistent reward and recognition.

We will also talk about the special case of how to deal with chronically low-performing employees at the end of this chapter.

Communicate, Communicate, Communicate!

If your employees are resistant because they don't understand the "why" behind your request that they do things differently, you will find that once you step up communication, they will get on board.

Connect to purpose. You will engage employees best by connecting back to their passion for delivering quality emergency care. In fact, most of the tools and techniques offered in this book are not "new things" that create "extra work." They are better, more disciplined, and more prescriptive ways to do things we already do. So be sure to position them that way.

If you are rolling out new tools and techniques that will reduce patient falls or improve patient outcomes, remind staff of why they went into emergency medicine in the first place: to deliver quality care. When you encounter resistance, ask the staff, "What's not right about this for the patient?"

If we call a discharged patient to follow-up and make sure he understands his discharge instructions, has filled his prescription, and is improving since his ED visit, this aligns with our ultimate goal of ensuring clinical quality outcomes and providing exceptional service.

If we give patients a time estimate of how long tests and procedures will take and explain the treatment plan (AIDET—See Chapter 7), our patients will experience less anxiety and be more compliant with the prescribed plan of care.

Use data to communicate. Whenever possible, support your reasons for new or enhanced behaviors with evidence-based data from the literature. You will find many studies cited in this book. This approach is particularly credible when communicating with physicians.

An example: One organization that Studer Group coaches recently asked its doctors to change the way they introduced themselves and explained procedures to patients. They developed a PowerPoint presentation that included more than 20 supporting references from the medical literature to make their case that AIDET (See Chapter 7) would engender more trust from patients, improve patient compliance to physician treatment plans, and reduce complaints and lawsuits. Suddenly, "soft stuff" like key words is not so soft!

Be transparent. Cascade communication consistently through all levels of the organization so everyone understands the external environment in the same way. If your organization is downsizing and layoffs are imminent, don't surprise people. As one CEO shared in an interview recently: "We send a message of confidence in our communications. A manager said to me, 'Thank you for telling me why we aren't filling that position. Now that I understand, I'm fine with it.'"

Ask your CEO to talk about external forces and resulting organizational changes at all employee meetings. Then bring it back to the department level. Many ED leaders use a "Flip-n-Tell" to capture key points at meetings they attend so they can communicate these accurately with staff in the department. They explain how what they learned will impact the ED specifically. The result is that everyone in the organization is aligned. They all understand the operating environment the same way. And they all share the same understanding of why the organization is responding the way it is.

Set clear expectations. When you communicate clear expectations, you align your vision as a leader with that of your employee and set her up for success to meet your goal. You can set expectations with objective, measurable goals (See Chapter 2), by role modeling new behaviors, with direct conversations that communicate your expectations, and through the use of paper-based competency assessments when learning new tools and behaviors.

Communicate progress to goals. Keeping your staff current on how the rollout of the new tool or tactic is going keeps everyone motivated and allows for quick course corrections. What is the compliance level in the department? What is the patient feedback?

What are the financial savings to the organization? In this book, you will learn how to collect feedback and measure results daily and monthly for sharing with staff on an ongoing basis.

Give opportunity for input. Once you announce to staff the what and why of a new tool or tactic, be sure to offer lots of opportunity for structured input. Instead of saying, "We need to reduce wait times. What should we do?" get their feedback on the functionality of a rough plan. Ask: "How realistic is the plan? How feasible? How else can we make it more effective?" This alleviates anxiety and improves buy-in

Train Staff with the Competencies
They Need to Succeed

Prescriptive training on new skill sets builds confidence and consistency as staff try on new behaviors that may feel uncomfortable at first. After training has taken place, it's important to have continued methods to validate and verify how well skills were learned as well as to give accurate feedback. As President Reagan once said, "Trust, but verify." This is the key to long-term success.

I coached one CFO who asked me, "What if we train all these people and they leave?"

And I responded: "What if we don't train them and they stay?" That is the greater risk to your organization.

You can train people all day long, but if you don't set clear expectations and require accountability, it won't matter...and it won't change your results. Throughout the following chapters, I will share recommendations for using direct observation, role modeling, and paper-based competency assessments to align leader and employee expectations and ensure accountability.

Reward and Recognize

I'll also be sharing more in future chapters about Studer Group's concept of "managing up"—or positioning others well— by harvesting opportunities for reward and recognition. You'll learn how this fits into the communication feedback loop and how to carry these "wins" in ways that create more buy-in and better results.

The fact is, rewarded behavior gets repeated.[3] That's the secret to generating momentum in your department when you roll out new tools and tactics for excellence. You will no doubt find that your high performing employees quickly see the benefits of what you are proposing and are eager to get on board. Then you can leverage this group for initial results, which will build more momentum.

Nearly all of the tools in the following chapters have built-in mechanisms to harvest what's working well and who can be recognized. In addition to sending personalized, handwritten thank-you notes (See Chapter 9), you can carry recognition verbally through real-time patient feedback.

Dealing with Low Performers

One of the main reasons we end up with barriers and resistance is the low performing employees we supervise. In fact, most barriers are either a result of broken processes or people who won't get on board. If it's a people issue, you'll need to address it to break down the barrier. Otherwise, you will never achieve the critical mass you need to move the department forward to long-term sustainable success.

The only thing that's worse than a good hire who leaves is a bad one who stays. Hiring right starts at selection by using tools and processes (e.g., peer interviewing, behavioral-based interview questions, and new employee meetings) that ensure employees are well-suited to both the position and the team they will work with.

Studer Group finds that most healthcare organizations have 8 percent low performers, 57 percent middle performers, and 35 percent high performing employees. If you're like many leaders, you will find that no matter how much you explain, train, and encourage your low performers, their main goal is to go back to the old way of doing things. That's why you should **spend most of your time re-recruiting your high performers and developing your middle performers.** They are the ones who will move performance in your ED.

While your aim should always be to coach low performers for better performance, you must also recognize it may be necessary to move them out of the organization for the benefit of the rest of the team if they do not improve. Studer Group recommends you hold highmiddlelow® conversations with each of these three groups on a consistent basis to move organizational performance.

What do low performers look like? Typically, they point out problems in a negative way, position leaders poorly, and may demonstrate little commitment to teamwork. They may be passive-aggressive or have little interest in improving their own performance (or that of the organization). When they come to work, they negatively influence the rest of the department or they may perform work with little regard for the behaviors of safety awareness. Sometimes low performers masquerade as high performers with strong technical or clinical skills. But their negative attitude or inability to be a team player gives them away.

Here's one litmus test: If this person resigned tomorrow, but both you and your staff were okay with it, you are dealing with a low performer.

One of the most important things to know about low performers is that they have serious staying power. Because they are convinced they can outlast any new initiative or leader, low performers can easily sabotage the effort of the whole group unless you take firm action with them.

Your goal is to re-recruit your high performers, coach your middle performers to a higher level, and take a strict "up or out" approach with your low performers.

> In our ED, nurses and techs work closely and collaboratively. Since we have 31 beds and an average daily census of 120 patients, each staff member's participation is critical.
>
> However, two of our low performers were techs. One had serious performance challenges... including refusing tasks and excessive computer use. The other tech had excessive absences. While both went through steps of corrective action, these techs did only the minimum required to avoid termination.
>
> As manager, I had tried to "rehab" these employees back to acceptable levels of performance and attendance. And yet, while this consumed much of my time, I was unsuccessful.
>
> Finally, I realized the impact these staff members were having on our top talent. I realized that other employees had to compensate for the presence of these low performers. It was an Aha! moment for me when I finally understood I could not force these low performers to change.
>
> At that point, I began to hold them accountable for their actions...the same accountability that I required of other employees. And in just a few weeks, they were managed out of the organization.
>
> The impact on the ED staff was impressive. Staff morale improved dramatically, and there was a sense of happiness at work, rather than the previous sense of dread when the low performers were

working. Once I replaced them with high performing techs, I watched our patient satisfaction scores
begin to show sustained improvement for the first
time in two years.

Larraine Yeager, RN, MSN
ED Manager, Presbyterian Kaseman Hospital,
Albuquerque, NM

How to Have a Conversation with a Low Performer

With low performers, be consistent in setting expectations and
consequences. Then follow through. If they continue to not meet
expectations, exit them out of the organization.

When you schedule a conversation with a low performer,
adopt a serious tone. Do not start out on a positive note. Use the
"DESK" approach:

D: Describe what has been observed

E: Explain impact of behavior

S: Show/tell what needs to be done

K: Know Clearly state consequences of continued same
performance

Follow-Up: Schedule follow-up conversation immediately
within improvement timeframe. (For more on how to conduct
highmiddlelow performer conversations, visit www.studergroup.
com/excellenceintheED.)

Embrace Creative Tension

Author Peter Senge[4] defines creative tension as the gap that exists when we hold a vision that differs from current reality. Or as Quint Studer says, it's the difference between current performance (where you are) and desired performance (where you need to be).

This tension, Senge says, can be resolved in two ways. You can either take action to bring reality into line with the vision—and move performance up—or you can lower your vision downward to release the tension (to allow people to feel more comfortable).

Creative people use the gap between what they want and what is to generate energy for change rather than to succumb to mediocrity. It is a tension of personal mastery and the source of all creative energy for innovation and process improvement.

As Quint explains, creative tension is not negative but it is often uncomfortable, which is why we must ask ourselves: *Is it the right thing to do? Even if I am uncomfortable?*

In his newest book, *Straight A Leadership: Alignment, Action, Accountability*, Quint explains that leaders in an increasingly difficult operating environment must continue to raise the bar by asking people to perform better so the organization can meet its mission. It's all about execution. Better execution means better care for our patients.

The reality is that change is here to stay. Volumes will continue to increase. We will continue to have more uninsured patients than we had a year ago. So embrace change.

At Studer Group, we believe that your best chance for success is to use the evidence-based tools in the coming chapters, because they have worked at hundreds of organizations to accelerate performance. If you verify and validate as you implement these tools and coach your staff to higher performance, the sky's the limit!

Key Learning Points: The Resistance Reality

1.   Ultimately, leaders are responsible for driving change. The sign of a true leader is his or her ability to develop a process for change, show others why they need to change, and to execute change.

2.   Why do staff resist change? A few reasons include the fact that it can seem risky; the purpose for change is not clear; leaders feel they lack the staff; they fear failure; or they lack the skill or the will.

3.   Once you understand the reasons for resistance, you can address them through strong communication, effective training, and consistent reward and recognition.

4.   One of the main barriers to moving organizational performance is the low performing employee. The only way to sustain long-term success is to take a strict "up or out" approach with them by setting clear expectations and consequences and following through. For best results, use the "DESK" approach to having a conversation with a low performer.

5.   Embrace creative tension: the gap between current performance and desired performance. While it can be uncomfortable, leaders must raise the bar and ask employees to execute at a higher level for the organization to meet its mission in an increasingly complex and challenging operating environment.

CHAPTER 2

Building the Case for Service

"There are no traffic jams along the extra mile."
—Roger Staubach

Emergency Departments are critically important to the health and well-being of Americans. In fact, in 2003, nearly 114 million visits were made to hospital EDs, more than 1 for every 3 people in the United States.[1]

And yet the pressures on EDs today are greater than ever before. Overcrowding is at the top of the list, with one recent study showing that large metropolitan EDs (serving more than 50,000 patients per year) bear the greatest burden. Representing just 17.7 percent of all Emergency Departments in the nation, these EDs accounted for 44 percent of all ED visits in 2007.[2]

As a result, 500,000 ambulances were diverted in 2007,[3] with potentially catastrophic treatment delays for those patients.

The role of the ED itself is changing. While 20 years ago the ED treated many seriously ill and injured patients, today it provides much more urgent and unscheduled care for Medicaid and uninsured patients who do not have access to primary care.

And yet, demand for a qualified workforce continues to outpace supply by leaps and bounds, with a shortage of more than one million RNs overall anticipated by 2020.[4] It has never been more critical to hire right and retain good employees.

Also, the reimbursement environment for hospitals has never been more challenging. With the Centers for Medicare & Medicaid Services' (CMS) refusal to pay for serious preventable adverse events (SPAE), hospitals can no longer afford patient falls or infections in the ED or inpatient units. Because resources are scarce, efficiency is key.

And, today's transparency means that consumers can comparison shop hospitals online to find out which ones have nurses and physicians who listen and explain best...those who are most likely to "always" treat patients with courtesy and respect. Due to HCAHPS (the Hospital Consumer Assessment of Healthcare Providers and Systems) and healthcare reform, we can anticipate that at some point reimbursement will align to hospital performance. Another reason why service is not soft stuff.

The good news: Providing excellent service is free. You don't have to put it into your capital budget. And because the ED experience has such an impact on the patient's perception of care as an inpatient, that good first impression is critical in the ED. It also provides a powerful way for the hospital to differentiate itself from competitors.

As the power of the consumer increases, it becomes mission-critical for EDs to listen and provide exceptional service to their patients.

What Patients Want

According to one report, the average amount of time a patient spent in the ED in 2008 was 4 hours 5 minutes.[5] Is it surprising then that lower patient satisfaction correlates with higher wait times? Or that keeping patients informed about delays is the top priority for improving the ED experience?[6] Over the past five years, the top three priorities for patients in the ED have remained the same:

Keep me informed about delays. Control my pain. And explain my plan of care.

Initially, patient satisfaction is about wait time. By reducing door to doc time, you will reduce risk in your ED and improve patient satisfaction. But over the long-term, you'll need to hardwire evidence-based leadership principles and practices to gain a true and sustainable marriage between service and quality.

For patients, there is little distinction between quality and service. They go together. A higher rate of patient complaints also correlates to greater malpractice exposure.

While patients expect clinical quality, they will differentiate you from other EDs based on service. If they have a bad experience, they hang on to it for years and years…repeating it to dozens of friends, colleagues, and acquaintances at work, at home, and at parties.

Your ED is not just the window to the community. It's also the front door to the hospital. As the entry point, you make an important first impression with patients that will—for better or for worse—make its way back to the rest of the community. Make a great one and that first impression will also drive referrals and market share for the rest of the hospital.

What will patients see when they open the door to your ED? Will they see that there's a long wait…that nurses seem harried and busy…or will they be greeted warmly, offered comfort items if there is a wait, and be updated frequently?

I recommend that ED staff "verbalize their value" and "narrate their care" as patients go through the ED experience.

What do I mean?

As a nurse in your ED, I can choose to approach you as a patient in two ways. I can go open the door to the lobby, hold on to the doorknob, yell out your name, and wait until you follow me back to a room.

Or, the minute I see you after I call your name, I can close the gap between us by walking over to you and greeting you and your family members. Then as we are walking back to the room together,

I can "manage up" the physician you'll be seeing as well as my own skill set by telling you a bit about my qualifications and those of your physician. I can also inform you that the physician will be in to see you within 15 minutes…and ask you if there's anything I can do for you while you wait. (For more on this, see AIDET in Chapter 7.)

In the same way, I can go into a patient's room, look at his wound site, check the IV, check the monitor and vital signs, ensure the side rails are up, and walk out of the room with a brief, "Everything looks fine" to the patient.

Or, I can say, "Mr. Andrews, I'm just taking your blood pressure. I see it's in a normal range now. That's great. Your wound site looks good and your lab tests should be back in about 20 minutes. I have the side rails up for your safety and it looks like everything is within reach on your bedside table. Dr. Johnson will be in in about 20 minutes to give you more information. Is there anything else I can do for you?"

It takes the same amount of my time. But by verbalizing my value and narrating care, I am also reducing the patient's anxiety and giving specific information that provides value. That patient will also be less likely to use the call light when I leave if they know what is happening now and what will happen next.

We find at Studer Group that EDs that earn high marks from patients on service and quality tend to do three things: They make a positive first impression. They give frequent and timely communication to patients. And they ensure a warm close with patients. In a high performing ED, quality and service go together and improve together. And none of this takes extra time.

It's not extra work. It *is* the work.

The best way to learn how to work smart and be efficient with your time is by using proven tools and tactics that have been tested in hundreds of organizations. We know they get results…and I'll be sharing many of them with you in the coming pages.

Evidence-Based Leadership^{SM}

Most of what we do in caring for our patients involves evidence-based practices. As Studer Group's Bob Murphy points out in *Managing Infection Control,*[7] we most certainly would not prescribe new medicine without an intensive scrutiny and evidence-based platform to ensure the best possible outcome. We would not perform medical procedures without proven evidence of their benefit. However, we often provide leadership based on limited evidence or how we've been taught by previous leaders or how it's always been done…which may not be standardized across the organization.

Typically, people believe they can provide strong leadership autonomously or without regard to standardization. Imagine the uproar if an ED nurse decided to give a medication without documenting it? Or started an IV without wearing gloves? What was acceptable 20 years ago isn't anymore. The standard of care is higher. It's imperative that leaders hold staff accountable to the standard of care and expected behaviors.

So why do so many of us wing it when it comes to leadership? Chances are that many of us were promoted into a leadership role without any training. If you have a great staff nurse, she'll probably eventually be a great charge nurse, the thinking goes. And yet, the skill set a leader needs to be successful is very different from the skill set we need to succeed in a staff position.

When I was first promoted to manager, I didn't know how to lead. It was uncomfortable. And when I felt discomfort because I didn't know how to develop a new staffing model or show the ED's financial impact to senior leaders, I'd notice myself gravitating back to clinical tasks where I felt confident and comfortable. I finally decided to invest in my own professional development and go back for my MBA, even though it was 10 years into my management career. I didn't lack the will. I lacked the skill.

It's okay if your leaders feel uncomfortable as they learn new leadership behaviors. We have to get comfortable with being uncomfortable as we grow our skill sets. The key is to provide mentoring.

Evidence-Based Leadership acknowledges that there are best practices proven to attain best results. As a result, leaders align goals across their organization and then align behaviors and processes. They hold themselves and others accountable along the way.

Figure 2.1

Evidence-Based Leadership℠ in the ED

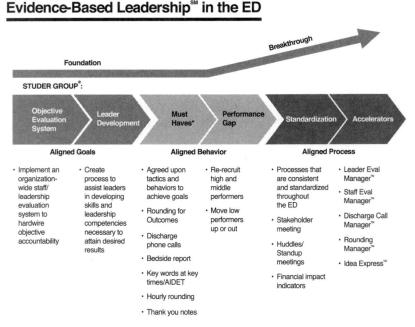

Evidence-Based Leadership aligns goals, behavior, and processes with tested tools and tactics that are proven to deliver breakthrough results.

The organizations Studer Group works with use an objective leadership evaluation tool to set and cascade all organizational goals and measure progress quarterly by department and individual. Because the goals cascade from the CEO to all leaders in the organization, everyone is aligned and accountable.

An aside: Quint Studer notes that most healthcare projects and initiatives come in over budget and late without achieving desired results. Why? Lack of alignment and accountability.

These leader goals reach staff as expected behaviors that align to the goals of the organization. So for example, if the ED's goal is to increase patient satisfaction from the 25th to 75th percentile, it means that ED staff will likely be making more discharge phone calls to patients and will commit to immediate bedding of patients and making hourly rounds in the reception area.

Once you've aligned goals and know where you're going, leadership development becomes the next key component. While many new leaders may have basic leadership skills, how frequently do they get training on how to develop a budget?

Or drive quality through measurable metrics? Or demonstrate return on investment and financial impact from changes implemented in the ED?

These are just a few of the skills that will create breakthrough performance in your department.

In its position statement on clinical nurse manager competency, The Emergency Nurses Association (ENA) notes that nurse managers work with many key stakeholders that are crucial to addressing issues of safe practice and safe care...not to mention cost efficiency, risk management, resource management, regulatory compliance, and more.

ENA defines core competencies in leadership development for nurse managers to include the ability to:

- facilitate conflict resolution;
- maintain, support, and encourage others with professional development;
- improve communication interdepartmentally;
- build collaborative relationships intra- and inter-departmentally;
- utilize negotiating skills;

- empower staff to participate in decisions; and
- promote change management processes.

What skills do leaders in your ED need? As Quint Studer says, "If organizations believe it's important to provide employees with the tools to be successful at their jobs, then the tools they should provide to leaders are leadership competencies."

Studer Group recommends that organizations provide leaders with 64 hours of training annually off-site at Leadership Development Institutes (LDIs). While conferences can provide useful training, a homegrown LDI that focuses curriculum on building the unique skills your leaders need to move organizational performance provides the best return on investment.

Since every ED may have different priority issues, a training curriculum developed by a committee at your organization will help you sequence training for best results. If your ED has high RN turnover, for example, then learning tools to improve employee selection and retention will be a critical first step to making gains in patient safety and quality.

If your service results are stalled, training your staff on how to improve effective communication with patients (e.g., AIDET and key words) might be in order.

If you're trying to improve quality of care by reducing your door to EKG times, you need to make sure there's a clear process in place to meet your targeted goal. You have to train your staff, set clear expectations, and audit and share results.

Leadership development training provides the link to learning how to set goals and metrics, identify performance gaps, and create accountability. Once you know where you are headed and have the skill set to get there, it's natural to give your staff the tools and tactics they need and begin to hold them accountable. Studer Group calls these the Must Haves®, which are designed to align behavior. You'll read about some of the most pertinent Must Haves for the ED—and how to hardwire them for long-term performance—in the coming chapters.

The second part of aligning behaviors is managing your performance gap. In addition to setting expectations for staff behaviors, this is your opportunity to re-recruit your high performers, coach your middle performers, and move your low performers up or out of the organization. This is the key to achieving breakthrough performance.

The last piece is aligning standardized processes. Once you have implemented the Must Haves, you'll ask: "What do I need to standardize to ensure these behaviors happen with every patient every time?" By standardizing key processes—like ED stakeholder meetings, for example—you'll hardwire key tools and tactics successfully.

Financial Impact

Frequently, the ED is seen as an expense to hospitals when actually so many things we do have a positive financial impact. Yet, we neglect to track and share them.

As you begin to implement some of the tactics in this book, they will have a direct positive financial impact on your ED. By increasing efficiency, for example, you have the opportunity to grow the volume of inpatient admissions. By implementing key words and AIDET with registrars, you can improve cash collections. By rounding hourly on patients, you will reduce falls (which are no longer reimbursed by CMS).

As ED leaders, it is our responsibility to show senior leaders the positive financial impact of what we do. It's also the best way to get the resources you need to move the department forward.

We don't get anything for free in the ED, right? If you go to your CNO and request more staff, what will she say?

No. Not likely.

But if, instead, you can show that a substantial net return on investment by reducing your Left Without Being Seen (LWOBS) patients by 4 percent over six months will net $720,000 in additional revenue, she may be more receptive to your request to hire that triage tech for the reception area. (Note: This is based on yielding an additional 1,440 patients per year in a 36,000 patient per year ED.)

Here are some additional examples:

- **Reducing ED turnaround time (TAT)**—A decrease in the overall ED turnaround time leads to higher patient satisfaction, fewer patients leaving without treatment, and a net gain in virtual beds

  If you reduce overall average TAT by 60 minutes in a 36,000 annual visit ED, you create room to see an additional 30 patients per day (virtual beds). If even half of those 30 patients are realized, the return on investment is dramatic. Based on an average reimbursement rate for an ED treat/release visit of $500 per patient, your ED earns $7,500 in higher revenue per day or over $2.5 million per year.

- **Reducing RN turnover**—If your ED employed 50 RNs and could improve employee satisfaction enough to reduce turnover by 10 percent (e.g., five RNs), you would yield $300,000 per year in savings. (This is based on an estimated cost of $60,000 per RN. However, the best way to calculate savings is to use the average RN salary and real staff numbers for your organization.)

- **Increasing number of patients registered per hour**— Let's say that your ED has a baseline of registering five patients each hour and sets a goal to increase that to eight patients per hour by better matching registration staff with census and by increasing accuracy. This would improve throughput times and revenue collection by 1) ensuring co-pays are collected and 2) ensuring every patient receives a full registration

If you add just one billable patient per day for one year—at an average reimbursement rate of $500 per ED treat/release patient—your ED would earn an additional $182,500.

- **Increasing volume**—Research shows that patients will tell others about a positive or negative ED experience. By using tactics in this book (e.g., rounding in the ED reception area, bedside report, discharge phone calls, interdepartmental communication tools) you can dramatically improve the patient experience as measured by faster turnaround times for tests and patient satisfaction scores. If higher patient loyalty grows ED volume by just 1 percent, that would yield an additional $180,000 in a 36,000 annual volume ED. (Calculations are based on 360 new patients, or 1 percent of a 36,000 annual volume ED at average revenue of $500 per patient.)

- **Reducing inpatient holding time**—A reduction in inpatient holding time of one hour per day would have the same impact as a decrease in overall turnaround time of 60 minutes. This would create room for the ED to see an additional 30 patients per day (virtual beds). If even half of those 30 patients were realized—at an average reimbursement rate of $500 per ED treat/release patient— the financial impact would be $7,500 per day or more than $2.5 million per year.

In closing, the best way to gain the resources you need in the ED is to demonstrate the positive financial impact and return on investment you deliver.

So build the case for financial impact. Demonstrate your fiscal responsibility. When you can show that there's a half million dollars of revenue still on the table that can be captured by reducing LWOBS another 4 percent, leaders will listen.

Getting the resources we need is our responsibility as ED leaders. When we can learn how to use objective data to state our case for financial impact, we will move the department forward.

Key Learning Points: Building the Case for Service

1. Pressures on the ED are greater than ever before. Overcrowding is at the top of the list. Caring for more Medicaid and uninsured patients, a workforce shortage, and an increasingly challenging reimbursement environment round out the list.

2. Today's transparency means consumers can comparison shop online to find out which hospitals have nurses and physicians who listen and explain the best.

3. What do patients want? To be kept informed about delays, to have their pain controlled, and to have their plan of care explained. These top three patient priorities have remained the same for five years as measured by many ED patient satisfaction surveys.

4. Patients don't distinguish between quality and service. They expect clinical quality, but will differentiate you from other EDs based on service.

5. You can "verbalize your value" and "narrate your care" to reduce patient anxiety and improve satisfaction without spending any extra time or dollars.

6. Evidence-Based Leadership acknowledges that there are best leadership practices that attain best results in the same way that evidence-based medicine does. This framework includes the use of an objective leader evaluation process to align and measure progress by departments and individuals and standardizes leadership development, behaviors, and organizational processes.

7. Successful ED leaders bring more resources to their department by measuring, tracking, and communicating the positive financial impact of indicators like reducing turn around time, holding time, LWOBS, and RN turnover as well as increasing volume and patients registered per hour.

CHAPTER 3

Connecting the Dots

"Creativity is the power to connect the seemingly unconnected."
    —*William Plomer*

At Studer Group, we use the term "connecting the dots" to link actions to the goals and values of the organization...to help others understand why we are doing what we are doing and engage their help.

And we use the Healthcare Flywheel® as a way to express the momentum for results on this journey.

At the center of the flywheel are purpose, worthwhile work, and making a difference. It's what has kept me coming back to the ED for the last 20 years. It's central and core to the work that we do.

Figure 3.1

Healthcare Flywheel®

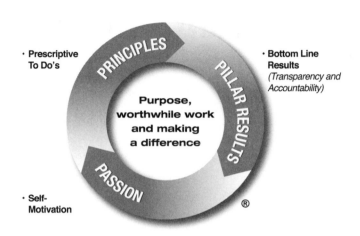

Passion is the upstroke of the flywheel. And, while there are times in our careers when passion is high or passion is low, the passion is what will move you to do the work that gets results.

The prescriptive "to-do's" are important. I can have all the passion in the world, but if I don't know how to channel that energy—how to use it—I won't get the results I want. These prescriptive tools are proven evidence-based tactics that will net you desired outcomes.

For example, consider hourly rounding…a tactic we'll examine more fully in Chapter 8. Each prescriptive behavior nets you a specific outcome. By asking patients about pain, we ensure they are comfortable…which reduces their need to use the call light. By asking if the patient needs to use the bathroom and ensuring everything is within reach, we reduce falls. If you don't use all the prescribed behaviors, you are leaving outcomes on the table.

But even if an individual's passion is low, these prescriptive "to-do's" will help. Many of us have felt frustrated and wanted to make changes but weren't sure how. The prescriptives provide the road map that will get desired results. This fuels momentum and motivation so each of us feels a sense of purpose, worthwhile work, and making a difference.

By helping staff connect back to that, we find that they respond in a powerful way.

I once heard Studer Group Coach Barbara Hotko explain how the Healthcare Flywheel is similar to the flywheel on a steam engine, which drives a train. She said, "When you listen to the sound of the engine, you can hear the push that starts the engine. Then as the engine moves, the train gains momentum, until the momentum is so great, it's difficult to stop. Some say it takes eight miles for a locomotive to stop."

That's how it works. By connecting to passion and purpose, we start the engine. When we inspire our employees to commit to very prescriptive "to-do's" (covered in Chapters 4-9), we begin to see some initial positive results. This turns the flywheel. Staff become more committed and satisfied. Results generate more results and spin the flywheel faster as we gain greater momentum on the journey to service and operational excellence...until behaviors are "hardwired^{SM}."

That means that prescribed behaviors are happening consistently with every patient every time. So even if leaders come and go at your organization, you will sustain the gains.

How to Turn the Flywheel

I'm sure you've heard it all before. Your organization announced that you'd be starting discharge phone calls, but there's no context around it.

Whenever we want our staff to do things, we need to connect back to why. We need to explain the plan and give them the road map and tools they need to succeed. Otherwise, they may get anxious. Be sure to share results to inspire more progress. Then they will spin their own flywheel and become more committed to the work.

So, you could say, "We're going to start making discharge phone calls to patients today." If you leave it at that, you'll probably encounter a great deal of staff resistance.

Or you could add the why: "Research shows that discharge phone calls are a best practice clinically. They reduce readmissions and save lives by ensuring our patients are following discharge instructions and doing well after their ED visit." Ask the staff, "How do you think we can get started?"

Most of us went into emergency care because we wanted to deliver great clinical care for patients. As a result, high performing employees will typically adopt new tools and practices that align with these values when they are presented in this way.

When staff are connected to purpose, they're willing to go through the pain of the change in order to provide better patient care.

We Do Sacred Work

Today in our ED, we witnessed both a tragedy and the amazing ability of humanity to shine. A little four-year-old girl who sold Chiclets gum on the border between Tijuana, Mexico, and San Diego, California, was accidentally run over by a car. When she was rushed to Sharp Chula Vista ED, physicians and nurses worked desperately to save her little life.

The professionalism, teamwork, and skill of the team led by Dr. Ali and Dr. Smith were amazing. Yet, the little girl didn't make it.

Soon her mother arrived, thanks to Immigration officials who bypassed regular paperwork and VISA regulations and even found a car seat to transport her and her infant. This mom had also been working among the cars with a baby papoosed on her back.

If you have ever heard the sound that a mother makes when she first learns of the death of her child, you know the sound of true agony and utter pain.

After being with her daughter for a while, someone heard the mother sob in Spanish that she didn't even have enough money to bury her little girl. The staff in the ED began passing an envelope to help this poor Chiclets-selling mother. Every nurse, every doctor, and every tech put everything they had in their wallets that day into the envelope.

When staff from RT, Security, Patient Financial Services, Pharmacy, and Radiology heard about the mother's situation, they too came to put money in. Patients and visitors who were lined up and down the busy ED hallways saw and heard the grief of this mother and insisted that they also wanted to put money into the envelope.

When Immigration brought the father, we were able to give him a hug and express our sincere sorrow for his loss. We told him that we were all crying with them and that we had a small expression of our great sorrow. He opened the envelope and he and the mother started to cry and expressed sincere thanks.

Although this little girl is no longer with us in this world, I will always remember her. She helped me see the beauty of humanity and reminded me why I love working in this hospital with such compassionate and talented colleagues and coworkers.

Joshua McCabe
ED Leader
Sharp Chula Vista Medical Center, Chula Vista, CA

The External Market: Is Your ED Unique?

I bet you're thinking: *What about me? It all sounds really wonderful, but my ED has special challenges.*

At Studer Group, we hear about many "special cases" as we travel around the country ...the reasons why this journey is so much more difficult for one ED than others.

We hear things like:

- We have more drug seekers.
- Our staffing shortages are more severe.
- We struggle more because our volume is so high.
- We have poor buy-in from Administration.
- We have to hold more patients than other EDs do.
- Our physical space is more limited.
- We have a higher acuity of patients.
- We have more recent nursing graduates than our competitor.
- We don't have good relationships with our physicians.
- Interdepartmental relationships with the Lab/Radiology aren't good.

Actually...we are not uniquely challenged. Even if you have one or many of the common challenges shared by many, many EDs on this journey, you can succeed.

Changes in the external operating environment have created a set of challenges that unite us more than those that differentiate us. ED visits are on the rise everywhere. The number of patients without insurance is also growing. Most of us will see an increase in volume because people have lost their jobs and insurance. Most of us will see sicker patients because they didn't go see their primary care physician.

The external environment—with more ED closures—will continue to put new pressure on all of us. And since it doesn't look like it's going to get any easier in the near future, Studer Group recommends you get ahead of the curve by implementing the Must Have® tactics in the chapters to come. By embracing the change, you'll be able to better manage the challenges you face.

Studer Group's five pillars and evidence-based leadership tools provide the framework you need to get ahead of the curve with breakthrough results you can sustain...whatever the circumstances in your ED now.

Frequently, we hear ED leaders say, "I'd love to do that, but I don't have the resources they have in those big EDs."

Or conversely, "I'd love to do that but we're a big ED. We can't turn on a dime like those smaller facilities."

In our experience, high performing EDs will relate—not compare—as they review potential tools, stories, and data.

If you put new tools and data in front of a high performer, he will say, "That's interesting. I wonder how we could make that work." High performers take things, tweak them, and adapt them to their environment. They know that if they wait for a perfect match, they will be paralyzed forever.

A middle performer will be willing to try, but might get stuck on the "how" to do it and resources needed. However, a low performing employee will say, "That will never work for us."

So relate—not compare—if you want to move your ED to higher performance. The best thing to compare is your ED's performance before you started using a new tool or tactic to once you've adopted it. Be willing to trial and test things.

Let's take an example. Say you're a busy 75,000 visits per year ED with 40 beds. You think your wait times are long because your volume is higher. The other ED in town has 30 beds and sees only 50,000 patients per year. *We could do better if we just had 10 more beds,* you think.

The reality is that reducing wait times is most impacted by how efficient you are at turning over beds, regardless of the size of your ED. Immediate bedding reduces door to doc time. In fact, at one ED I managed prior to Studer Group, we implemented a rapid cycle improvement project called "WOW: Wipe Out Waiting" that reduced patient cycle times by over 30 percent and doubled cash collections while improving patient satisfaction to the 90th percentile in "wait-related" questions.

How did we achieve it? We closed the registration window and redesigned the registration process. A security guard greeted people arriving in the ED and directed them to complete a brief patient information form. A triage nurse then completed a brief assessment in a private area while a registration clerk simultaneously constructed a patient account number and chart. If a bed was open in the ED treatment area, the patient would proceed directly to a room after the registrar verified brief demographic information, got consent for treatment, and arm-banded the patient. While patients waited for physician-prescribed treatments and therapies, registration clerks obtained and verified insurance information and collected co-pays. In short, using parallel processes significantly shortened waiting times.

It's also not always about needing more beds or more staff. It can be about how you delineate work to maximize each staff role in the department.

In a position statement on the role of delegation by the emergency nurse in clinical practice settings, the Emergency Nurses Association recommends that emergency nurses use their education, expertise, and ability to make delegation decisions based on an assessment of potential risk of patient stability, degree of critical thinking required, predictability of outcome, the degree of patient-family interaction needed, and the impact on timeliness and continuity of care.

While things like the overall assessment of the patient, planning, evaluation, triage, and coordination of care are clearly the role of the nurse, he may delegate things like taking vital signs, performing EKGs, applying a splint, or transporting non-monitored patients. The goal is to maximize the role of both your licensed and unlicensed personnel in the ED to drive efficiency.

Another opportunity is to maximize efficiency by matching your staffing model to your patient flow. You can do this by reviewing arrival times on a 24-hour basis to determine staff-to-patient ratio needs. If, for example, you get busy at 10 or 11 a.m. and stay peaked until 11 p.m., with quieter times around 2 or 3 a.m., you can taper your staff accordingly. For example, you can have a nurse come in from 3 p.m. to 3 a.m. instead of 7 p.m. to 7 a.m. to better cover your peak times and match your patient flow.

If you truly find you need to add additional FTEs, make the case effectively. For example, you can show that if you reduce your LWOBS rate by just 1 percent, you will increase revenue for the department with a return in real dollars. If you really want to be successful getting that FTE, pilot the proposed staffing changes for 90 days before you ask. Then show real data on positive financial impact achieved.

The Five Pillars

Whatever your goals, Studer Group recommends using a balanced approach...because the "fire hose" approach just never works.

That's where the five pillars come in.

The five pillars provide the foundation for setting organizational goals and direction for service and operational excellence in the ED. They also provide consistency over time that allows an organization to resist new "flavor of the month" programs and create focus with priorities, particularly when there are just too many things on our plate.

Most organizations use service, people, quality, finance, and growth as the five pillars, although some add community as a sixth. And under those pillars, we use key metrics to measure the things that drive excellence in our ED.

One of the best things about the evidence-based leadership tactics we will be reviewing in upcoming chapters is that they deliver benefits and wins under multiple pillars. For example, if you implement hourly rounding in your ED reception area (Chapter 4), you will see improvements under the service pillar (higher patient satisfaction) and under the quality pillar (improved clinical outcomes when you catch changes in patient status more quickly). Because these patients have been informed about delays and offered comfort items during rounding, they will be more willing to wait for treatment. When your LWOBS rate drops as a result, you'll see higher revenue under the finance pillar. Volume will also improve under the growth pillar as great service begins to drive word-of-mouth referrals. When your employees feel that sense of purpose, worthwhile work, and making a difference, your employee retention will rise under the people pillar.

And higher employee retention—which really means lower employee turnover—correlates directly with better clinical outcomes. (See below.)

Figure 3.2

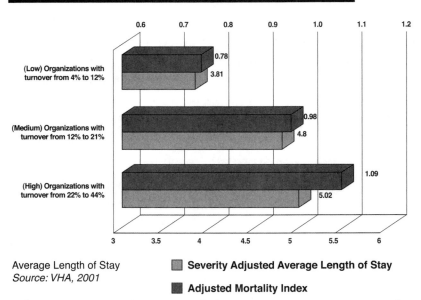

Lower Employee Turnover Means Better Patient Care

In this VHA study, organizations with the lowest employee turnover also had the lowest average length of stay and lowest adjusted mortality index.

Studer Group finds that organizations that use the five pillars to align goals create and sustain results. They better understand their own goals and their current position with respect to those goals. Also, since all leaders are evaluated against established metrics under each pillar, it provides a framework for the evaluation process, meeting agendas, communications, and work planning... keeping the organization balanced in both its short- and long-term objectives.

In short, the pillars ensure our priorities are focused and our vital resources are appropriately distributed so that we get the long-term results we are seeking.

Figure 3.3

The Five Pillars Deliver Bottom-Line Results

Service	Quality	People	Finance	Growth
• Increased patient satisfaction • Decreased patient complaints • Reduced claims • Reduced malpractice expense	• Improved clinical outcomes- decreased patient falls • Decreased door to provider times • Decreased AMAs • Decreased unscheduled 48-hour returns • Reduced medication errors	• Reduced turnover • Improved employee and physician satisfaction • Reduced vacancies • Reduced agency costs • Reduced overtime • Reduced physicals and cost to orient	• Increased revenue • Increased upfront collections • Decreased left without treatment rates • Improved payer mix	• Increased volume • Improved word of mouth • Improved market share

But you have to have the "why." That's why the flywheel is so important. While we all know what's right to do and *want* to do these things, we need a balanced approach with a road map to actually achieve them. When we marry the prescriptive "to-do's" to mechanisms for accountability and provide a feedback loop, we move forward and get in front of challenges. This provides the systematic approach we need to succeed.

Unfortunately, the things we did in the ED 15 or 20 years ago just won't get us there in today's operating environment. Instead, we know that high-performing leaders will commit to a disciplined evidence-based approach with prescriptive tactics that have demonstrated they deliver consistent results.

The reality is that we can't afford to leave the success of our ED to chance. The external environment is just too unstable. By using a methodical approach over time, you can drive an effective culture of excellence in your ED. That's how you weather the storm. In Section 2, you'll learn about three foundational Must Have tactics to move your ED performance in 90 days, so let's get started!

Key Learning Points: Connecting the Dots

1. Connecting the dots means linking actions to the goals and values of the organization to help others understand the why and to engage their help.

2. Studer Group uses the Healthcare Flywheel as a way to express the momentum for organizational results. At the center of the flywheel is our individual desire for purpose, worthwhile work, and making a difference. By tapping into employees' personal motivation, we inspire them to commit to some very prescriptive "to-do's," which turns the flywheel and delivers initial results. Results create more momentum as the flywheel spins faster, generating more results until they are "hardwired" (i.e., prescriptive and expected behaviors happen with every patient every time).

3. Many EDs feel they are unique and different in some way (e.g., more drug seekers, worse staffing shortages, poor physician or interdepartmental relationships, higher volume). But what we know is that those with breakthrough results relate—not compare—because evidence-based leadership tools have been proven to work in all types of EDs.

4. Changes in the external operating environment have created a common set of challenges that makes us more alike than different.

5. Studer Group recommends a five pillar approach —service, people, quality, finance, and growth—to provide the foundation for setting organizational goals and direction for service and operational excellence in the ED. They align goals and behaviors, and standardize processes, such as meeting agendas, communication, and work planning.

Three "Must Have" Tactics to Move Your ED in 90 Days

CHAPTER 4

Rounding for Outcomes

"The greatest leaders aren't necessarily the ones who do the greatest things. They are the ones who inspire others to do the greatest things."
— *Ronald Reagan*

What Is Rounding for Outcomes?

Rounding for outcomes is the consistent practice of asking specific questions one-on-one of staff and patients to obtain actionable information. It's Evidence-Based Leadership℠ at its best. In fact, Quint Studer in his bestselling book *Results That Last* says, "Rounding for outcomes enables a leader to play offense, not defense."

In my experience, **leader rounding on staff is the single best way to raise employee satisfaction and loyalty and ultimately attract and retain high performing employees.** It helps employees feel they have purpose, worthwhile work, and are making a difference. It improves employee satisfaction by providing that which is important to them.

In the same way, rounding on patients improves clinical outcomes, promotes patient safety, and increases efficiency in the ED.

In both cases, rounding for outcomes seeks to build relationships; learn what is working well; harvest "wins"; identify areas for process improvement; repair and monitor systems; and ensure staff have the tools and equipment to do their jobs safely each day. Because it achieves all this, it's a foundational strategy and the first tactic to implement as you work to remove barriers to an excellent ED experience.

Four Types of Rounding

In the Emergency Department, there are four types of rounding: 1) leader rounding on staff, 2) leader rounding on patients, 3) rounding in the reception area, and 4) staff rounding hourly on patients, which will be discussed in Chapter 8.

Leader Rounding on Staff

The number one reason we round on our staff is to build the relationship between the supervisor or manager and that employee. Leader rounding reduces employee turnover. That's because the number one reason employees leave an organization is because they have a poor relationship with their supervisor.[1]

Leader rounding delivers on this desire very specifically. And since happy employees lead to happy physicians and patients, it's the number one action you can take to raise employee, physician, and patient satisfaction.

When you round on your staff, you will stay close to what is working well in the ED, who should be recognized for exemplary work, and what opportunities exist for improving efficiency with systems and processes. You'll also learn what functional tools and equipment they need to do the job.

Because you're more connected with your staff, they will feel they have a voice at the table. You can validate positive staff behaviors so they become hardwired, manage up high performers, and identify trends and opportunities for improvement.

You'll even find that you're able to minimize the voice of the low performer by creating a more stable and cohesive voice for the whole department.

How Often to Round on Staff

Studer Group recommends these guidelines for rounding on staff:

- Up to 40 direct reports: Round once per month (two per day).
- 41 to 80 direct reports: Round once every other month (two per day).
- Greater than 80 direct reports: Round once per quarter (two to three per day.)

If you have a large number of reports, you can also share the rounding responsibility with your supervisors to maintain the monthly rounding contact. Of course, leaders should always communicate to staff that their input is welcome at other times as well.

Questions to Ask During Leader Rounding

The number one reason employees leave a position—39 percent—is because they have a poor relationship with their supervisor.[2] What staff want in a leader is approachability, to work "shoulder to shoulder," tools and equipment to do their jobs well, appreciation, efficient systems, and opportunities for professional development. [3]

You can respond to these drivers of employee satisfaction by asking your staff these questions:

1. *What's working well today?* Consider opening with a relationship-building question (e.g., "I hear your daughter graduates tomorrow. What are her plans?"). Always begin with the positive. It's important to help staff remember that good things happen daily. Another way to ask is: "What's the best thing that happened this week?"

2. *Is there anyone I should recognize for doing great work?* Ask staff to be specific. When you round on staff, but receive a general comment such as "Saul's great!" you need to dig deeper. Say, "Tell me more. Why is Saul great?" Then deliver the win. Say: "Saul, Lynne really appreciated that you came in and covered that sick call so they didn't have to work short last night. Thank you!" This allows you to carry the compliment to a coworker or physician to strengthen the relationship. Not only do they feel good about the leader who has given the compliment, they feel great about their coworker for recognizing them. This turns the flywheel, building momentum for better service, teamwork, and higher clinical quality.

   Rounding is a wonderful way to learn about the amazing things your staff are doing that would otherwise go unrecognized. Remember, what gets recognized gets repeated!

3. *Are there any systems or processes that need improvement today?* You might hear that the CT scanner will be down for several hours, which will require communication to staff and patients. However, you might also learn that the new self-scheduling process is working well. Having this information allows you to adjust and respond to both issues in real-time.

How is that new process working? If you've recently implemented a new process, this is your opportunity to find out more. If you've just implemented discharge phone calls, for example, you can ask: "What is working well with the discharge phone calls?" "Do you have the forms you need to track the calls?" "Who's doing a great job making the calls that I should recognize?" "What have you learned from making the calls?"

4. *Do you have the tools and equipment you need to take care of patients safely today?* This helps you identify barriers that can be immediately addressed. You might hear about simple fixes (e.g., "I've been looking for a blood pressure cuff/ thermometer/pulse oximeter cable for 20 minutes!"). There may be times the barrier is more complex (e.g., "Can we add a field on the electronic health record?") and may require more time for follow-up. What's important here is to provide staff expected timeframes for completion. Let them know you will be providing updates as more information becomes available.

5. *Is there anything I can help you with right now?* You build credibility with your team when you are willing to assist when necessary. Maybe your nurse has four patients to dis charge and is feeling frustrated. A quick win is to say, "I've got a few minutes. Let me do one for you." A little goes a long way when trying to build trust, confidence, and col laboration. A bonus: You'll have an opportunity to spot check the patient's experience of care

This is also a good time to discuss things, such as professional development (e.g., "I wanted to talk to you about applying for your certified emergency nurse certification" or "Let's talk about a development plan to orient you to the charge nurse role"). High performers want opportunities for development and will appreciate your making this a priority.

New leaders might also want to ask, "What's the one thing I can do to be a better leader?" This shows approach ability and willingness to accept feedback.

Track Results from Rounding: Use a Rounding Log

Rounding logs are not optional. They are critical to the long-term success of rounding. In fact, Studer Group coaches frequently tell leaders they coach on rounding, "If you want incremental results, then don't use a log. If you want sustained results that accelerate progress, then logs are a Must Have® to help you move faster."

As a leader, your staff are your customers in the same way patients are the customers of your staff. They deserve to hear back from you when they bring up a request, issue, or concern, so write it down on the log.

And when you write things down, connect the dots for staff by explaining why you are writing it down. You don't want them to think something unpleasant they said is going to be placed in their file. Say, "I'm going to take a few notes so I can follow-up on this for you."

Rounding logs also reveal key trends. When you hear that 10 of your staff are having trouble with Radiology, for example, you need to follow-up with that department leader. Items from rounding logs also roll up into your Stoplight Report (see page 55) so you can report back accomplishments and the status of requests to staff.

Figure 4.1

Sample: Leader Rounding on Staff Log

Tool	ED Rounding on Staff Log
How is it used?	To document feedback from rounding on staff To verify behavior is hardwired
Measures of Success	Increase in employee satisfaction Decrease in turnover
Tips for Implementation	The following information should be documented • Date • Employee • Items for follow-up • Compliance with rounding parameters
Ease of implementation 1=difficult and 5=easy	3
Notes	Validate competency of leaders rounding on staff to optimize desired outcomes

Department:_____ **Date:**_____

Items to address during rounding:
- Personal Connection/Relationship Building
- What's working well
- Staff and/or physicians for recognition (who/what/why)
- Systems that need improvement
- Tools and equipment to do your job
- Tough Questions

Name	Date	Notes

Total Number of Staff:_____ **Total Number Rounded On:**_____ **% Compliance:**_____

To download a full-size version of this sample, go to the *Excellence in the Emergency Department* resource page at www.studergroup.com/excellenceintheED.

Capture Rounding Outcomes with a Stoplight Report

When I started rounding, I noticed that sometimes my staff would forget the 29 things I did for them last month based on their requests. Even though we'd hired two nurses, changed physician hours, and bought extra thermometers, one person really wanted those new gurneys right away.

The stoplight report captures all requests during rounding and codes them green, yellow, or red so everyone knows where their item stands. Green means, "You asked. We listened. It's done. We accomplished it."

Yellow means, "We're working on it but it might take a little time." Items coded yellow (e.g., hire two technicians, implement a self-scheduling process, etc.) should be completed within 90 days.

Red means, "I'd love to have it too, but it's not going to happen right away." If you know the request is not going to happen, do not put it in red. Rather, have a crucial conversation with your staff about why it can't happen. Otherwise, you create "we/they" in your organization, as in "I requested additional staff on the stoplight report but management won't let me hire them." Good leaders avoid "we/they" and tackle tough questions directly.

Good leaders also redirect and focus staff on the things the team can impact rather than allowing them to spend time on those things that are out of their control. They also share the stoplight report with their leaders to escalate issues that need attention to improve systems and processes.

Figure 4.2

Stoplight Report

Wins From Rounding   Month_____

ACCOMPLISHED		PENDING		FUTURE	
ITEM/PROCESS	DATE	ITEM/PROCESS	DATE	ITEM/PROCESS	DATE
Purchased two new thermometers	10/16	Hire two staff positions	By 11/15 in interview process now	New parking structure	Next year

To download a blank full-size version of this template, go to the *Excellence in the Emergency Department* resource page at www.studergroup.com/excellenceintheED.

Financial Impact: Leader Rounding Reduces Employee Turnover

Leader rounding on staff dramatically improves employee satisfaction for higher employee retention. When you lose an experienced nurse, there is an emotional and quality cost to the Emergency Department. You may also risk losing other nurses if the individual who leaves now encourages other colleagues to join them at the new hospital.

Consider this: **If you reduce RN turnover from 20 percent to 10 percent on a staff of 50 RNs at a cost of $60,000 per RN, the additional five RNs you retain will save your ED replacement costs of $300,000.**

Tip: When you track and measure financial gains from lowering turnover in your organization, always use actual costs at your organization for best accuracy of savings. Some organizations may have an annual RN salary that is either lower or higher than the $60,000 national average. Other organizations I know recommend using a blended rate for better accuracy of true costs, by including salary loss and advertising costs as well as training and overtime costs.

Figure 4.3

Evidence-Based Tactics Reduce Employee Turnover

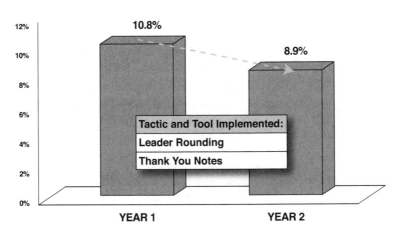

Source: Ohio Based Healthcare System, Admissions: 39,067, ED visits: 185,279, Beds: 1,009, >6,400 employees

By implementing leader rounding on staff and thank-you notes, this organization reduced employee turnover by 1.9 percent in just one year, retaining an additional 12 employees for a savings of $720,000.

Leader Rounding on Patients

The purpose of leader rounding on patients is to: 1) ensure we are providing the best possible quality care to the patient; 2) harvest reward and recognition for our staff; and 3) identify trends and opportunities for improvement. Leader rounding on patients also validates that staff are executing the behaviors that we've asked them to do to improve the patient experience.

And, it enables you to hear firsthand the amazing things your staff do for your patients every day to put them at ease and make them more comfortable.

Once I heard a nurse in a busy ED take an extra moment to give a patient an empowering choice when starting her IV. "Where's your secret vein?" he said. The patient visibly relaxed as she pointed him to the best spot and responded, "They never have any luck with the veins in my left arm, but this one in my right wrist always works."

I bet some of your high performers often dim the lights and offer a cool washcloth to patients with migraine headaches. Are we thanking our staff for showing such compassion to the patients' personal needs?

Once leaders are consistently rounding on staff, they should begin rounding on patients as quickly as possible or at least within 90 days. Here's why: When you round on patients, you'll harvest good reward and recognition and uncover coachable moments to bring back to your staff.

By beginning leader rounding on patients soon after implementing rounding on staff, you will be better able to identify and address habits that staff may have picked up when learning these new behaviors so you can change them.

In the same way, I recommend that each time you put a new process in place, you round on patients to check the experience from the patient perspective. This allows you to make any needed course corrections quickly and provide positive feedback to your staff that will further strengthen the behaviors.

Questions to Ask When You Round on Patients

The goal here is for you as a leader to validate that the staff are using the behaviors that will support patient priorities. You may also choose to focus on one or two trends or opportunities you have identified in your patient satisfaction survey results or discharge phone calls. (See Chapter 5 for more about discharge phone calls.)

Another goal is to keep the rounding encounter from three to five minutes. You want to have a brief but meaningful conversation with the patient and drill down in any needed areas. It's also important to do an environmental safety check to make sure the room is clean, the side rails are up, and ensure the patient has access to the call light and necessary items are within reach. Rounding on patients also offers an opportunity to provide comfort items, such as ice, blankets, pillows, water, or a chair for a family member.

A conversation might go something like this:

Open with:
"Hello, Mr. Johnson. My name is Sue and I'm the nurse manager here in the Emergency Department. I am making my patient rounds to ensure we are providing you very good/excellent care (use survey words) during your stay. I just want to ask you a few questions. It should take less than five minutes. Is now a good time?

Ask specific questions. Some areas where you can drill down include:

- *Pain.* "Our goal is to make sure we are managing your pain well. Are the nurses asking you to rate your pain on a 1 to 10 scale?

  "Is your nurse asking you your name, date of birth, and checking your armband for safety before giving you any medications or treatment?

" I see you received medication at 10 a.m. Has the nurse or physician been back to re-assess your pain since then?"

- *Plan of care.* "We also want to keep you informed during your visit. Has the nurse or physician updated you on your plan of care and what will happen next?"

"Did the nurse tell you when the lab results would be back?"

"Do you know what you're waiting for?"

Ask: "Is there anyone who has been particularly helpful to you today that I can recognize?"

When the patient says, "My nurse Dan says he has been a nurse here for 15 years. He is really experienced!" you as a leader can feel confident that your nurse is "managing themselves up" with a strong introduction. (See The Five Fundamentals of Service in Chapter 7.)

Maybe a patient tells you, "Dan said I'm really lucky to have Dr. Johnson for my cardiologist. He says I'm in great hands." Then you know Dan's effectively managing up physicians to help reduce patient anxiety and ensure smooth hand-offs.

Ask: "What is one thing we can do to improve?"

Then close with: "Do you have any questions I can answer for you?" "Is there anything else I can do for you before I go?"

When you leave the patient, give the staff immediate feedback. Close the loop by complimenting the employee the patient named: "Angela, Mrs. Martin really appreciated your attention to her pain levels over the last four hours."

It's also important to give a global acknowledgment to staff at the desk: "In all 14 rooms I rounded on, every patient said they were asked their name, date of birth, and their armbands were checked before they received medication. Thanks for doing such a great job keeping our patients safe today." This drives up the positive emotional bank account with your staff.

Coaching staff is just as important as giving reward and recognition to hardwire new behaviors. For example, if the fourth room you rounded on had two-day-old information on the whiteboard, speak to that nurse about it directly.

Rounding on patients in this way provides an opportunity to validate and reward behaviors you as a leader asked staff to do. And by being in the patient room, you'll often have the opportunity to see the special touches your high performers use when doing them...like the nurse who isn't just keeping the whiteboard current but also includes the words "proud to work here since 1995" right under his name.

Remember, your rounding on patients is not complete until you have given staff feedback—for better or for worse—and filled out your rounding log.

Figure 4.4

Sample: ED Leader Rounding on Patients Log

Parameters
- 25% of treat and release patients
- 100% of patients holding for an inpatient bed

Key Word (excellent, very good, completely satisfied)
Area of Focus (behavior that is being hardwired)
Example: Hourly rounding on patients to address Pain, Plan of Care, Delays (PPD)

"Our goal is to provide you with very good care which includes rounding on you each hour to manage your pain, review your plan of care and keep you informed. How well are we doing?

Patient	Type	Feedback on Area of Focus Working Well (WW) or Needs Improvement (NI)	Staff	Recognize	Coach	Notes

Total Number of Treat & Release Patients: _____ Total Number Rounded On: _____ % Compliance _____

Total Number of Patients holding for a bed: _____ Total Number Rounded On: _____ % Compliance _____

Name: _____ Date: _____

To download a full-size version of this sample, go to the *Excellence in the Emergency Department* resource page at www.studer-group.com/excellenceintheED.

Patients Notice: Capturing the Wins

On a Sunday afternoon at about 4 p.m., I dropped in at the ED to see how the staff and patients were doing. I started in the waiting room where Reggie was triaging. She told me about Mrs. Scott, a 62-year-old African American woman who presented with chest pain and syncope. The patient was so impressed that she could have her EKG completed at triage and that she was then moved directly to a treatment room.

When I rounded on her in the room, I shared my card and introduced myself as the director of nursing for the ED. I told her that our goal was to provide her with very good care and asked if there was anything I could do to make her more comfortable. By glancing at the whiteboard, I was able to manage up Dr. Shand (her physician), Choban (her nurse), and Brian (her patient care technician).

Then Mrs. Scott said, "What is going *on* around here?"

"From the time I hit the door, the staff introduced themselves, explained what the plan was for my care and told me when the tests would be back!" She went on to further explain how impressed she was with Dr. Shand coming to her bedside and sitting at eye level to explain everything.

When I left Mrs. Scott's room, I was able to give immediate feedback to Dr. Shand, Choban, and

Brian. They were thrilled. In fact, their excitement was contagious. Other members of the team asked if I would also speak with their patients that day. They too wanted to hear what their patients had to say!

Deborah C. Stamps, MS, RN, GNP, NE, BC
Director of Nursing, Emergency Services &
Diagnostic Imaging
Rochester General Health System, Rochester, NY

Figure 4.5

Leader Rounding on Patients Increases Patient Satisfaction

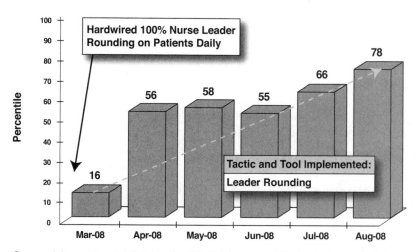

Source: Arizona Hospital, Total beds: 355, Employees: 4,000, Admissions: 10,188

This organization increased patient satisfaction from the 16th to the 78th percentile in just five months after hardwiring leader rounding on patients.

Rounding in the Reception Area

If you're like many ED leaders, you might call the ED reception area the ED "waiting room." But does this send the right message to patients?

When I coach Emergency Departments, I urge leaders and staff to think of their ED as less like a waiting room and more like their living room at home. When you have a guest over, for example, would you want them to feel like an inconvenience or as an invited guest? In the ED, it's important that patients feel welcome. We want to make sure our living room is clean and that we don't leave our guest unattended for long periods of time without company. There needs to be dialogue.

So, I ask you: Is the thought of rounding in your reception appealing? No.

Are people afraid? Yes!

In fact, if your security guards are even afraid to go out there, you know you need to round!

But here's what's in it for you:

- Reduced patient anxiety
- Fewer interruptions to the triage nurse and other staff members
- Greater patient confidence and trust because you will reassure them that it's okay to wait. As a result, you'll reduce the number of patients who leave without being seen.

Staff know it's going to be painful. But here's what we know at Studer Group: It's going to be painful only in the short-term.

Once you begin rounding consistently in the reception area, you and your patients will enjoy a quieter and calmer environment where patients are better prepared to receive care. And your staff will enjoy a less hostile working environment.

In one ED where I began working as the ED director, the reception area was a war zone! Nobody could get anything accomplished due to the constant interruption of patients checking back at the triage desk. Beginning hourly rounding in the reception area was a high priority for me.

Although the staff knew we needed to do it, the hard part was figuring out how. We got staff together and told them what we were going to do, and asked them, "What's the most natural model we can use to make it work?" As a result, they came up with the model we implemented.

While the triage nurse had primary responsibility for rounding in the reception area, we also engaged the security guards. We committed to using "close the gap" behaviors each time staff came to the lobby to get a patient. So, for instance, when staff called a patient name, they would also make eye contact and walk towards him or her. When they spoke to them, they made it a goal to also speak to two additional people...perhaps a family member or another waiting patient. In this way, we touched more patients with each contact that we made.

Consider the following true scenario reported in a nursing journal[4]:

A young woman approaches the triage desk for the third time in the last hour. "I can't wait any longer...I'm in so much pain. I'm too sick to sit here. How much longer do I have to wait?"

The triage nurse rechecks the patient while calmly explaining the situation in the ED. The patient sits back down, but 10 minutes later, comes back to the desk and says, "That's it. I'm leaving. I've been waiting for over two hours and you have taken other people ahead of me and they don't look sick. What do I have to do? Die out here before someone will take care of me?"

Patients like this one leave without treatment in Emergency Departments every day, putting us at risk both legally and financially. And even though it may feel like a relief to staff in an overcrowded ED when some patients are leaving, these risks to the organization can be great.

The average ED loses at least 2 percent of patients—and revenue—because patients choose to leave before getting treatment. If we can keep just two to three extra billable patients—who would otherwise leave without treatment—each day for a year, that adds an additional $219,000 to $328,500 to your organization's bottom line. (Note: Assumes an average reimbursement rate of $300 per treat and release ED patient.)

Figure 4.6

**Rounding in the Reception Area
Reduces ED Left Without Being Seen**

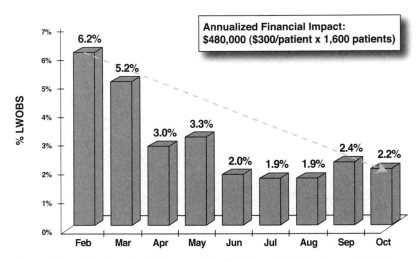

Source: Texas Hospital, Admissions: 12,705, ED visits: 40,000, Employees: 1,611

This Texas hospital realized an additional $480,000 in just eight months (while under full construction) by reducing their LWOBS rate 4 percent by hardwiring rounding in the reception area.

When we round in the ED reception area, our goals are to:

1. Show care and concern for patients

2. Keep them informed about delays to reduce the number of patients who leave without treatment

3. Reassess the patient's status to ensure safe clinical outcomes (This supports the ED's ability to meet the Joint Commission's standards regarding timely reassessment of patients.)

4. Improve patient satisfaction. Patients and families are more willing to wait if they receive hourly updates. They feel more comfortable and less anxious if they know we haven't forgotten about them.

I know one ED that received a letter from a patient complimenting them on the six-hour wait! The patient said that hourly rounds by staff kept him informed...and that made it a much more positive experience than when he had been to the ED the year before and waited for hours with no updates.

Hourly rounding in the reception area of the ED is the first and fastest way to effectively begin rounding on ED patients. In Chapter 8, I'll explain in-depth how to do it in your treatment area as well.

Who Rounds on Patients in the Reception Area?

While the triage nurse owns the process, EDs that Studer Group coaches use charge nurses, registration clerks, security, chaplains, case managers, ancillary staff from other departments (such as Radiology), and even senior leaders to help round in the reception area. It's a team sport!

Everybody wins when patients are kept informed. Nurses at the triage desk are no longer interrupted continuously by patients, families, and visitors. Staff are not confronted by angry patients when they open the door to bring the next patient back. Patients are more relaxed and can focus on receiving care.

Here are some examples of key words to use when rounding in the reception area:

Goal: Keep patients informed about delays. The triage nurse can say:

- "Our goal is to provide you 'very good' care while you are in the Emergency Department." *Reassure the patient that it is safe for them to wait.*

- "There is a wait right now, but we will be checking on you about every hour to keep you informed and make sure that you are doing okay. Please let me know immediately if you feel worse and I will reassess you." *Manage up the physician.*

- "Is there anything I can do for you right now?"

Goal: Keep patients informed about delays. These key words can be used when staff are conducting reception area rounds.

- "Mr./Mrs. Jones, I'm _____ (*name*) and I am just checking on you to see if you are doing okay. I apologize for the wait. Thank you for your understanding. Is there anything I can get you right now?" *Manage up the physician and offer comfort measures—warm blanket, water, assistance to bathroom.*

Goal: Provide a positive experience when escorting patient from reception area to treatment area. Staff can say:

- "Mr./Mrs. Jones?" *Move toward patient to meet/assist them.* "Good morning. I'm _____ (name) and I will be taking you to your room so that you can see the physician now. *Greet family as appropriate, manage up staff and physician and assist patient with orientation to room, need to undress, etc.*

Goal: Provide a positive experience when escorting patient from reception area to a hall bed. Staff can say:

- "Mr./Mrs. Jones?" *Move toward patient to meet/assist them.* "Good morning. I'm _____ (name) and I will be taking you to the treatment area so that you can see the physician now." *Greet family as appropriate, manage up staff and physician.*

"I know your goal is to see the physician as quickly as possible. I don't have a private room for you just yet, but I am going to place you here in a hall bed so that the physician can see you and get your care started. Please know that we will move you to a private room as quickly as possible and will make every effort to maintain your privacy needs while you are here. If you are more comfortable waiting in the reception area until a private room becomes available, just let me know." *Nearly all patients will be happy for the opportunity to see the physician more quickly and will not resist hall bed placement when these key words are used.*

To download a full-size version of these sample key words, go to the *Excellence in the Emergency Department* resource page at www.studergroup.com/excellenceintheED.

Keep a Reception Area Rounding Log

Just as leaders use a log when they round on staff and patients, those who round in the reception area should also use a log. (See sample on page 71.)

This is a 24-hour log with pre-printed times and a place for staff to initial and write comments. When staff round hourly, they can note things like "reception area is empty," "25 people waiting," "all families updated," or "no security guard today."

The manager then reviews the log for trends (e.g., We're always busy between 3:00 p.m. and 5:00 p.m.) and compliance with rounding. Is the log filled out 100 percent of the time? Or is it always incomplete in the late afternoon because staff are too busy or one individual doesn't use the log?

Leaders should also review results and trends from the log daily during daily huddles or stand-up meetings with staff. Share the wins, trends, and opportunities frequently so they understand the value of rounding in the reception area.

Figure 4.7

Sample: ED Reception Area Log for Hourly Rounding

Date:_____

TIME PERIOD	STAFF INITALS	COMMENTS
7:00 AM		
8:00 AM		
9:00 AM		
10:00 AM		
11:00 AM		
12:00 PM		
1:00 PM		
2:00 PM		
3:00 PM		
4:00 PM		
5:00 PM		
6:00 PM		
7:00 PM		
8:00 PM		
9:00 PM		
10:00 PM		
11:00 PM		
12:00 AM		
1:00 AM		
2:00 AM		
3:00 AM		
4:00 AM		
5:00 AM		
6:00 AM		

Staff signature:_____ **Staff signature:**_____

Staff signature:_____ **Staff signature:**_____

Staff signature:_____ **Staff signature:**_____

To download a full-size version of this hourly rounding log, go to the *Excellence in the Emergency Department* resource page at www.studergroup.com/excellenceintheED.

Key Learning Points: Rounding for Outcomes

1. Rounding for outcomes is the consistent practice of asking specific questions one-on-one of staff and patients to obtain actionable information.

2. There are four types of rounding in the ED: Leader rounding on staff, leader rounding on patients, rounding in the reception area, and hourly rounding in the treatment area (Chapter 8).

3. Studer Group recommends leaders round on two employees per day as a guideline. Rounding typically takes less than five minutes per individual.

4. Begin rounding on patients within 90 days or sooner after you have begun leader rounding on staff.

5. Use a rounding log and follow-up. There are three types of rounding logs included in this chapter (for leader rounding on staff, leader rounding on patients, and leader rounding in the waiting room/reception area). The rounding log is critical to your success because it lets you keep notes on what you learn and harvest wins. Be sure to communicate trends and opportunities with staff on a daily basis.

6. Any rounding is better than no rounding! Don't let lack of time or unfamiliarity with the process deter you from rounding.

CHAPTER 5

Discharge Phone Calls

"Discharge phone calls save lives."
—Quint Studer

Why Bother?

It's not unusual for staff to resist making discharge phone calls to patients in the beginning. In a busy Emergency Department, making calls can seem like just one more thing that we don't have time to do! As a leader, you can address staff pushback by role modeling making the calls and always connecting back to purpose. Ask: What's not right about it for the patient?

After working with hundreds of leaders around the country, I know that it takes only one call that saves a patient's life to make an individual a believer in discharge phone calls forever.

Discharge phone calls improve clinical outcomes, increase patient satisfaction, and decrease costly and unnecessary return visits to the ED as well as re-admissions to the hospital. Consider these facts: In one study of 400 patients, almost one in five patients reported an adverse event post-discharge. Forty-eight percent of those events were preventable![1] In an August 2005 follow-up study,[2] researchers found that of those patients who reported adverse events in the original study, 71 percent were significant, 13 percent were serious, and 16 percent were life-threatening. Since most EDs admit only14 to 18 percent of their total patient volume, more than 80 percent of patients will return home after their ED visit.

And yet, one study found that 65 percent of discharged patients said no one talked to them about managing their care at home.[3] Many patients will be confused or misunderstand their discharge instructions. They may not fill their prescription because of cost, concerns, or questions. In fact, according to an article in the February 2003 issue of *Annals of Internal Medicine*, the authors noted that confusion or misunderstanding about discharge is one of the top eight patient dissatisfiers and frequently leads to non-compliance with physician discharge orders, particularly around medication administration.[4] As a result, the authors noted that it's crucial to manage the first 72 hours after discharge to minimize adverse events and improve clinical outcomes. In Studer Group's experience, ED discharge phone calls are most effective (to demonstrate care and concern, improve clinical outcomes, and decrease re-admits) when made within 72 hours of discharge.

Having personally made hundreds of discharge phone calls, I've found that these calls—just two to three minutes each—deliver so many benefits. First, they demonstrate our empathy for the patient and his family by asking, "How is your pain?" "Did you get your prescription filled?" "Do you understand your discharge instructions?" Patients are so grateful that we cared enough to call and check on them.

This perception is particularly powerful if the physician who cared for the patient in the ED is the one calling. And if the physician can't call, there's still an opportunity to manage up the physician by saying, "Dr. Jones asked me to call and check on you." Patients appreciate that their doctor cares about them. We also consistently find that discharge phone calls improve clinical outcomes and allow staff and physicians to validate that the patient understood his or her discharge instructions and is doing well in the home environment.

Discharge phone calls also provide an opportunity to harvest reward and recognition for your staff and find out what went well. It's an opportunity to let the patient know they will soon be receiving a satisfaction survey and that you want to ensure they received very good care. It's also an opportunity for service recovery if the patient expresses concerns about his or her ED experience so they remain loyal to the organization.

When I first started making calls, I would make them from the main nursing station in the ED so staff and physicians would see firsthand that I was committed to making the calls; that they took just two to three minutes each; and that I was hearing a lot of positive feedback from the patients.

Discharge Phone Calls Save Lives

I will never forget one of the first discharge phone calls I made many years ago. We had just rolled out the process in the ED and since I was the ED director, I was really striving to be a "first mover" and role model for my staff. During my 12-hour clinical shift the day before, I had cared for a 19-year-old Laotian college student who presented with a chief complaint of fever and having "the worst headache of his life." The ED physician did a full work-up on this young man, including a battery of lab tests, a CT scan of his head, and a lumbar puncture. Several hours later, after some IV fluids and pain medication, the patient was discharged home with a diagnosis of viral meningitis and a referral to a primary care physician.

When I called his dorm room early the next morning to check on him, his roommate told me he was sleeping and seemed to be fine. When I learned that the roommate would likely return after his morning classes, I called back. His roommate said he was still sleeping.

I asked him to please wake my patient and see if he would come to the phone to talk with me. I listened helplessly as his roommate laid down the phone and tried repeatedly to wake his room-mate up in an increasingly loud tone of voice. When he finally re-turned to the phone, he was frantic.

"I can't wake him up!" he said. "He's all sweaty and he looks like he has the chicken pox!"

As you can imagine, my heart sank into my stomach at that moment. I asked the young man to stay on the line while my ED unit secretary called 911 and dispatched an ambulance to their lo-cation. Within about 30 minutes, the patient arrived unconscious and unresponsive, with a fever of 103.8 degrees Fahrenheit. He was covered with petechiae. We immediately instituted isolation pre-cautions, intubated and stabilized him, and admitted him to the Intensive Care Unit. I informed his roommate of his condition, and he quickly made contact with his family in Laos.

Later that day, the infectious disease physician in charge of his care stopped by the ED and asked who had made the discharge phone call to the patient. I told him I had.

He said, "Well, that phone call saved his life. He would have been dead by 5:00 p.m."

In all the time that has passed since then, I will never forget how I felt at that particular moment. Several of my staff and phy-sicians were there when the physician made these comments and actually gasped out loud after hearing his words. Time seemed to stop for several minutes and I literally felt paralyzed by that news. **What if I hadn't made the initial call? What if I hadn't been persistent and called back?** Eventually the moment passed, and like any good ED nurse, I returned to caring for my patients through the end of the shift.

But the story didn't end there. The next day, while I was in my office, I received a call from the ICU that the patient's family had arrived and wanted to talk with me. I quickly made my way to the ICU waiting area and greeted the patient's mother, father, and younger brother. Through broken English, they expressed their gratitude to me for "saving their son's life" and thanked me for making the phone call to check on their son.

Over the next week I saw the family frequently and shared in their joy as their son improved and was able to be discharged home from the hospital with minimal complications. I'll never forget his smile and words of thanks as he was wheeled out to his car. That moment is forever stored in the "fond memories" section of my brain. It was also the moment I made a personal commitment to making discharge phone calls forever. Having had this experience, how could I do otherwise?

Before You Begin Making Calls

Similar to rounding for outcomes (described in Chapter 4), discharge phone calls also provide an opportunity to harvest reward and recognition for staff and physicians, learn about the patient's perception of care, gather process improvements, and identify trends.

For example, when you make discharge phone calls, patients will tell you who your high performers are. You'll also learn where your opportunities for improvement lie. For example, Press Ganey's Priority Index for Emergency Departments consistently shows that patients' top priorities are: 1) managing pain well; 2) understanding their plan of care; and 3) being kept informed about delays. If you consistently hear patients say that staff were rude or rushed or they didn't understand what to do when they went home, you can address these trends.

But be prescriptive. In the same way you wouldn't casually put in a new chest pain protocol, be methodical about implementing and hardwiring tools (e.g., rounding for outcomes) that address these concerns.

If you haven't hardwired leader rounding on staff and patients before beginning discharge phone calls, guess what happens? You will hear lots of complaints on the calls. By addressing the things that staff and patients tell you need to be fixed *during* the patient experience, you will get more wins during the follow-up calls.

Remember, though…a complaint is a gift. You don't have to micromanage every complaint, but when you notice a trend during your calls (e.g., many patients saying that they weren't kept informed of what was going on during their stay), follow-up to hardwire and standardize better processes that drive clinical quality. If you address the top three patient concerns, you'll find that you receive fewer informal and formal complaints.

Prior to implementing discharge phone calls, it is crucial to hardwire leader rounding on staff and patients. Consistent and daily rounding on staff and patients provides the foundation necessary to be successful with discharge phone calls. It also ensures you have an effective accountability system in place to address followup concerns or complaints you identify during discharge phone calls.

How and When to Make the Calls

Which patients will you call? What questions will you ask? How will you document results for tracking purposes?

The long-term best practice goal is to **attempt to call 100 percent of eligible patients discharged to home, reaching 60 percent of patients within 72 hours after discharge from the ED.** Why? Research shows[5] that more than 90 percent of adverse events will happen within the first 72 hours of discharge. Ineligible patients include those who were admitted or transferred, psychiatric patients, or those who expired in the ED. Organizations using this best practice goal typically see initial results in 60 to 90 days. Patient satisfaction is higher and both formal and informal complaints in the ED are lower.

How to make the calls: One easy model to follow is to have the night shift prepare the list of eligible patients to call and pass this on to the day shift each morning. The day shift charge nurse distributes the calls evenly among all staff members and physicians who will be working that day and evening. Each person is responsible for completing their assigned calls during their shift. Calls are typically made between 8 a.m. and 8 p.m. using a standardized question template that focuses on key questions to ensure consistency. (See sample template on page 83).

Ask staff to attempt each call three times. Decide within your organization if employees will leave a message when they can't reach a patient. If so, what will they say?

I recommend leaving a message such as:

"Good morning. This is Stephanie calling from XYZ Hospital for Mr. Jones. Please return my call at 555-1212. If I am not available, please ask to speak to the person in charge. Thank you." This lets patients know that you care, while still respecting HIPAA privacy requirements.

Documentation is crucial to the overall success of discharge phone calls and must be considered an "always" behavior when making calls. Successful EDs utilize a standardized question template that staff use to document at the time of the call. The manager collects and reviews these daily for the purpose of sharing wins (e.g., "Karen, your patient Mrs. Jakowski was so grateful for your responsive and thoughtful care yesterday") and opportunities with staff and physicians (e.g., "Two patients say they waited three hours without being informed about delays. Let's make sure we are rounding every hour to avoid this concern in the future").

Documentation also allows you to identify trend issues that need resolution or course corrections. If, for example, patients are complaining that they are waiting too long from arrival in the ED to receiving pain medicine, you can re-educate staff about using the pain protocol more consistently. You might do a pain audit by pulling charts and determining the average wait time for patients between arrival and pain intervention. (Remember: Pain is the number one reason patients come to the ED.)

Leaders should share results daily in huddles or stand-up meetings (read more about these tactics in Chapter 9) and discuss findings weekly with their management team to determine appropriate courses of action. Many EDs use Studer Group's new system to automate the process, improve trending, clinical interface and reporting capabilities, and accelerate the hardwiring of discharge phone calls.

Who Makes the Calls?

I find that in high performing EDs, all nurses and physicians participate in making calls daily. This creates awareness and buy-in from the team of caregivers about the strengths and opportunities that exist in the department. The calls also build camaraderie as callers harvest and share recognition and compliments from patients with others.

ED support staff can also make discharge phone calls. Many EDs have successfully utilized greeters, volunteers, access/registration staff, ED technicians, unit secretaries, and staff on light duty. We know from experience that patients are "wowed" when they receive a discharge phone call. Remember—any call is better than no call!

When using non-licensed staff, it is critical to provide adequate training, use a standardized question template, and ensure there is a clear process for them to follow if the patient needs to be referred to a nurse or physician for follow-up. Many EDs have the shift charge nurse on point to take immediate calls that require clinical follow-up.

Figure 5.1

Sample: ED Discharge Phone Call Question Template

To be completed at time of discharge-

1. In order to provide _____care, we would like to follow-up with a phone call in the next few days.
   May we have your permission to contact you?   Yes   No

2. Please verify your phone number: _____

3. What is the best time to reach you at that number? Morning Afternoon Evening

4. Do you have any questions or concerns before you are discharged?

Follow up call

Attempts to contact: Date   Time   Initials
                        Date   Time   Initials
                        Date   Time   Initials
Introduction

My name is _____. I am a nurse calling from _____.

Dr. _____ asked that I call to see how you are feeling.

Comments: _____

1. Are you having any **pain**? Yes, Pain Level_____   No   N/A
   How are you managing your pain?   Medication Heat/Ice Elevation Other

2. Have you filled your prescriptions (if applicable)?   Yes   No (review)   N/A

3. We want to ensure you understood your **plan of care.**
   Did your discharge instructions answer all of your questions? Yes   No (review)

4. Do you feel you were kept informed during the **duration** your stay? Yes   No (review)

   Comments _____

5. Have you made a follow up appointment? Yes   No (review)

Closing

6. We always want to make sure our patients receive _____care.

   May I ask how your overall care was? _____

7. What is one thing you feel we could do to improve? _____

8. Are there any individuals whom you would like me to compliment for the care they

   provided? _____

Thank you note sent   Yes   No

Further Follow up   Contact MD   Contact Charge Nurse   Contact Nurse Mgr Other

Signature of RN_____   Date/Time _____

Track Your Calls

Just like with rounding for outcomes, tracking results is integral to success. If you are using a manual system, ask staff to place their completed discharge phone call logs in a central place at the nurse's station once they're complete.

At the end of the day or next morning, the manager or charge nurse can review the tracking logs for trends and opportunity and enter key data into a central spreadsheet.

Figure 5.2

Sample: ED Discharge Phone Call Trend Report

Date	Discharge Census	# of Calls Attempted	% of Calls Attempted	# of Patients Contacted	% of Patients Contacted
01/01/09	118	60	51%	40	34%
01/02/09	147	60	41%	42	29%
01/03/09	137	60	44%	39	28%
01/04/09	138	60	43%	38	28%
01/05/09	127	60	47%	35	28%
01/06/09	133	60	45%	40	30%
01/07/09	117	60	51%	42	36%
01/08/09	143	60	42%	36	25%
01/09/09	139	60	43%	35	25%
01/10/09	144	60	42%	22	15%
01/11/09	149	60	40%	21	14%
01/12/09	153	60	39%	45	29%
01/13/09	130	60	46%	35	27%
01/14/09	134	60	45%	29	22%
01/15/09	143	60	42%	36	25%
01/16/09	135	60	44%	42	31%
01/17/09	168	60	36%	35	21%
01/18/09	166	60	36%	32	19%
01/19/09	155	60	39%	30	19%
01/20/09	158	60	38%	28	18%
01/21/09	147	60	41%	32	22%
01/22/09	166	60	36%	42	25%
01/23/09	133	60	45%	43	32%
01/24/09	135	60	44%	40	30%
01/25/09	157	60	38%	27	17%
01/26/09	132	60	45%	25	19%
01/27/09	147	60	41%	36	24%
01/28/09	140	60	43%	47	34%
01/29/09	133	60	45%	50	38%
01/30/09	146	60	41%	25	17%
01/31/09	131	60	46%	32	24%

By logging the number of calls attempted and percentage contacted, you'll learn how well the process is working and who's making calls. Higher contact rates correlate with better results. In Studer Group's experience, **EDs will begin to get results when they attain at least a 60 percent contact rate.**

Return on Investment

It's human nature to ask, "What's in it for me?" So leaders should be prepared to answer this important question before implementing discharge phone calls. I believe the answer to this question is tied to our values. If I know that doing something in a prescriptive way will consistently produce a positive outcome for me and my patients, my values will dictate that I do this. You will also get better staff buy-in if you role model making the calls.

Those high performing EDs that are calling 100 percent of eligible patients discharged to home and reaching 60 percent of them are experiencing a number of positive outcomes:

Patient satisfaction is higher. Discharge phone calls are a "wow" factor for patients. In our experience at Studer Group, discharge phone calls typically increase patient satisfaction 25 to 30 percentile points. In fact, Hackensack University Medical Center in Hackensack, NJ, tested the impact of ED discharge phone calls by adding a question to their patient satisfaction survey: Did you receive a follow-up phone call the day after your visit? The results: Patients who received the call were far more likely to recommend the hospital (98th percentile) than those who did not receive a call (56th percentile).

Figure 5.3

Discharge Phone Calls
Improve Likelihood to Recommend

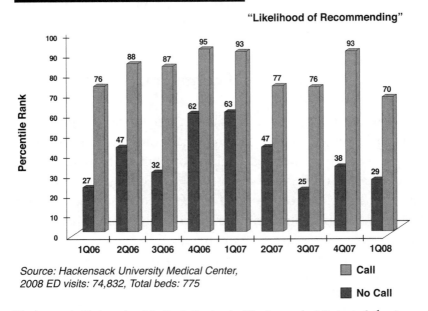

"Likelihood of Recommending"

Source: Hackensack University Medical Center,
2008 ED visits: 74,832, Total beds: 775

Hackensack University Medical Center in Hackensack, NJ, tested the impact of discharge phone calls on ED patients by comparing those who received a call to those who did not. Consistently, those who received the call were far more likely to recommend the ED than those who did not receive a call.

Increased understanding of discharge instructions and lower re-admits. In the Hackensack study above, there was also a difference of seven mean points in how well patients understood discharge instructions—which represents the difference between ranking in the bottom quartile or top decile of this vendor's ED national database. When physicians and employees make the call within 72 hours of discharge, they can assess the patient's progress at home and quickly determine if a patient is in distress or needs immediate intervention. They provide an additional opportunity for the patient to ask questions about medication and discharge instructions.

This in turn increases patient compliance with physician instructions for better clinical outcomes. As a result, there are fewer return visits to the ED.

Higher employee engagement. In my experience, staff who make discharge phone calls feel strongly connected to purpose, worthwhile work, and making a difference. They tell me that they feel a sense of doing what they went into emergency medicine to do and have a greater sense of confidence that their patients are receiving quality clinical care and understanding the physician's discharge instructions. (Carol, an ED staff nurse at a large ED in the Pacific Northwest recently told me that, "Making discharge phone calls is the best part of my day. It confirms that what I do is making a difference for my patients.") Additionally, by harvesting compliments of staff who did a great job for patients, you create an upward spiral of momentum that delivers greater teamwork and even higher performance.

Fewer patient complaints. If you've hardwired leader rounding and key words at key times (see Chapter 7), you will most certainly hear fewer patient complaints when you make discharge phone calls. In fact, fewer complaints on the calls will help you to validate that the changes you are making during the patient experience are working. But remember: A complaint is really an opportunity. It gives you a chance to identify trends that drive clinical quality and patient satisfaction. By addressing concerns and complaints on the call, you can also provide service recovery to the patient.

Greater patient loyalty and market share. Have you ever been at a party and found someone anxious to share their bad ED experience with you once they learn you work in an ED? If you ask them when this occurred, they'll tell you it was 10 years ago. They just won't let it go! And they'll tell everyone they know. Discharge phone calls bring positive word of mouth that inspires patient loyalty and grows your volume. And not just from patients...but from your staff who will tell people out in the community how proud they are to work in your ED. That's right...you can feel proud to wear your name badge in the grocery store!

With results like these, how can you afford not to make discharge phone calls? Having worked with many leaders, I know that once you make the calls and experience the value, you will never go back. Discharge phone calls provide a quick return on the investment of your time. Within 60 to 90 days, your staff will be happier; you'll have fewer complaints; and there will be more reward and recognition to share with your staff.

In fact, of all the Must Have® tactics to move ED performance, discharge phone calls offer some of the quickest results and perhaps the most immediate personal gratification. You'll learn things you can implement immediately to positively impact the next patient's experience. No need to wait for a survey to come back to tell you how to get better!

Key Learning Points: Discharge Phone Calls

1. Discharge phone calls improve clinical outcomes, increase patient satisfaction and market share, reduce complaints, and decrease costly and unnecessary re-admissions. They save lives.

2. Hardwire leader rounding on staff and patients first, before beginning discharge phone calls, to ensure success.

3. Discharge phone calls take on average two to three minutes each. Also, you can leave a HIPAA-compliant message.

4. Best practice is to attempt to call 100 percent of eligible patients discharged to home, reaching 60 percent of eligible patients within 72 hours after discharge. Organizations that use this best practice typically see results in 60 to 90 days.

5. The night shift can prepare the list of patients for the day shift to call each morning. The day shift charge nurse distributes calls evenly between staff and physicians who will be working that day and evening.

6. Documentation is crucial to the success of the discharge phone calls. Use a standardized question template at all times. Use the tracking log to track calls and identify trends.

7. In high performing EDs, all nurses and physicians make calls daily. If they are trained, support staff can also make calls, to include greeters, volunteers, registration staff, ED technicians, unit secretaries, and staff on light duties. Any call is better than no call!

CHAPTER 6

Bedside Shift Report

*"Good communication doesn't have to be extensive.
Simple and clear goes a long way."*
—John Kotter

Why Is It Important?

The short answer: patient safety. Bedside shift report is also an excellent way to build employee teamwork, ownership, and accountability.

The truth is, thousands of patients are cared for every day in U.S. Emergency Departments, resulting in thousands of shift changes and thousands of opportunities for error. According to the Institute of Medicine's report *To Err Is Human: Building a Safer Health System*, between 44,000 and 98,000 people die in U.S. hospitals each year due to preventable healthcare errors.[1]

Even greater are the numbers of preventable errors that do not result in death, but lead to acute or chronic illness, injury, and/or disability. Financial costs from errors are also substantial and include lost income, reduced productivity, increased healthcare costs, and inflated health insurance premiums.[2]

The ED is a high-risk environment in which additional safety factors must be considered. The National Quality Forum identified these as:

- multiple individuals involved in the care of a single patient;
- patients with high acuity illness or injury;
- rapid healthcare decisions under severe time constraints;
- high volume of patients and unpredictable patient flow;
- barriers to communication with patients, families, and other healthcare professionals; and
- interactions with multiple types of diagnostic and/or treatment technology. [3]

The bedside shift report tactic also responds directly to a number of the Joint Commission's National Patient Safety Goals, including Goal 1 ("Improve the accuracy of patient identification" because we check the patient armband and ask the patient his name and birth date as identifiers); Goal 2E ("Improve the effectiveness of communication among caregivers: managing hand-off communications," with particular attention to assuring the opportunity for asking and responding to questions); and Goal 13 ("Encourage patients' active involvement in their own care as a patient safety strategy").[4]

Bedside Shift Report Works

Everyone in the ED knows that shift changes are the times when patients use call lights the most. They wonder where everyone is! So you'll be happy to know that bedside shift report also reduces call lights dramatically.

Of course we know that every ED nurse already reports on his or her patients. But when we bring the report to the bedside, we gain an opportunity for real-time exchange of information between the oncoming and offgoing nurses as well as the patient.

Bedside shift report is increasingly becoming recognized in the industry as a best practice. In fact, I know one organization—a recent winner of the prestigious National Quality Forum Award—that actually invited Joint Commission surveyors to round with nurses as they did bedside shift report during their visit. Surveyors praised them highly for the high level of patient involvement and thorough exchange of knowledge during the bedside report process.

Manage Up, Transfer Trust, and Build Confidence: What's in It for Staff

While it all sounds simple, staff may be resistant to this process for any number of reasons. But here's the really wonderful thing: Bedside shift report drives staff ownership and accountability.

How many times have you heard staff comment: "You should see the way the night shift left their rooms!" or "The IV is dry. His sheets are wet and there are two full urinals on the mayo stand!"

In the beginning, bedside shift report offers opportunity for staff to have real-time conversations. If I go into the room and see that the last nurse has left it in disarray, I can say, "Kim, why don't you empty the urinals while I check the patient and update the whiteboard?"

If I, as a staff nurse, understand that bedside report is an expectation and I'm clear that someone is going to be checking both my patients and my rooms, as well as verifying my charts, then I'm going to be more likely to make sure everything is in order prior to that shift change.

You might hear staff concerns that it will "take too long," or "I don't have time! I've got four patients to pick up from three nurses!" or "They'll ask us too many questions."

I know I did, when I first implemented bedside shift report. The reality though is that nurses will be with the patient for three to five minutes while they physically check the patient, update the whiteboard, and do an environmental check (e.g., Is the IV patent? Are the side rails up? Does the patient have the call light within reach?).

In fact, bedside shift report actually buys the oncoming nurse a little time. Because it's a quick physical check on the patient, he can ensure the patient's room is in good condition and the patient is safe and then check on other patients. And it's also a warm hand-off...allowing the patient to say goodbye and thank the nurse who has cared for her during her stay.

Bedside shift report is a wonderful way to mentor newer nurses in your department too. It's good discipline for someone to review their documentation, physically see their patients, and review their assessments, medication therapy, and environmental factors every 12 hours. Who knows? A new nurse could be so busy focusing on her clinical skills that she forgets to think about patient comfort measures.

However, **before attempting to implement this process, be sure you have already hardwired leader rounding on staff and leader rounding on patients** to ensure that your staff are engaged and that you have a process in place to obtain feedback from patients. (See Chapter 4.)

If you want implementation to go well, planning is everything. At Studer Group, we recommend you use AIDET^{SM} (See Chapter 7 for more about **A**cknowledge—**I**ntroduce—**D**uration—**E**xplanation—**T**hank You) and SBAR (page 99) to communicate effectively during bedside report.

And, before you start, you'll also want to discuss with staff why you are implementing bedside shift report. Review the process and gain agreement. And finally, verify outcomes through leader rounding on patients. In the end, I can assure you that the benefits of bedside shift report clearly outweigh the barriers. By standardizing communication around shift change, caregivers feel more prepared to answer patient questions. The offgoing nurse can also give updates on plan of care and share which orders are still pending.

What's in It for Patients

As mentioned previously, the most compelling reason to commit to bedside shift report is patient safety. In 2005, a Joint Commission analysis found that 70 percent of sentinel events were caused by communication breakdowns, with half of those occurring during hand-offs.[5]

In fact, my own mother—a retired nurse—who has had multiple ortho surgeries related to her osteoarthritis, has experienced two significant medical errors over the years. One of them occurred just prior to a shift change and could have been identified and corrected quickly if a bedside shift report process had been in place.

Sometimes it takes a personal experience for us to remember that this is really about our own loved ones getting safe care.

The key to successfully hardwiring bedside report is to implement processes that clearly define the responsibility from one caregiver to another, standardize the communication process, and allow for an interactive exchange between the parties involved. Bedside shift report decreases the potential for near misses through a transfer of responsibility and trust and by using standardized communication.

It also increases patient involvement in their plan of care in these ways:

- Patients see and hear from the team of professionals who are providing their care. As a result, they feel more comfortable asking questions or voicing concerns.
- Patients are reassured that everyone is getting the necessary report about what is going on with them.

- Patients feel more informed about their care, which makes them less anxious and more compliant with the plan of care.
- Patients are more satisfied because they know that things are being monitored throughout the shift.
- Patients know who their nurse is on every shift.
- Bedside shift report reduces the perception that "no one is around" during shift change (when sentinel events are more likely to occur).

Figure 6.1

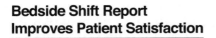

**Bedside Shift Report
Improves Patient Satisfaction**

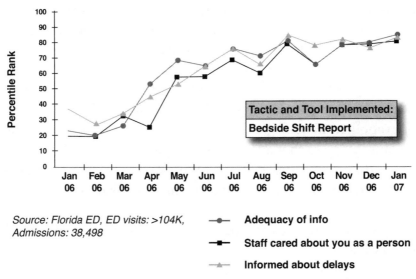

Source: Florida ED, ED visits: >104K, Admissions: 38,498

This Florida ED improved patient perception of care—based on three survey indicators—dramatically over the course of one year by using bedside shift report.

How to Implement Bedside Shift Report

The short version: Bedside shift report is meant to be fast. Before entering the patient's room, the oncoming nurse will look at the chart, go over medical history, treatments, and anything pending while at the desk…just like he normally does. Then the offgoing and oncoming nurses will go to the bedside together where the offgoing nurse manages up the oncoming nurse and introduces him using AIDET. (See Chapter 7.)

The oncoming nurse's role is to ask the patient his name and date of birth, and to check the armband for safety and introduce himself. He should update the whiteboard in the room and double-check pumps as well as all IV meds for accuracy and the patient's safety.

The Steps

1. **Prior to bedside shift report, advise and educate the patient that it will be occurring.** I know some EDs that even provide patients with a letter to explain and manage up the process.

   > **Sample Letter to Patients About Bedside Shift Report**
   > *To our patients:*
   > *At (hospital name), we conduct "Bedside Report" to keep you better informed about your plan of care, medications, tests, and progress while you are here. This involves the nurses doing bedside reporting, in your presence, at each shift change to ensure proper communication of all-important information and to introduce you to your new nurse.*

> *In the event that you have visitors in your room at the time of Bedside Report, or anytime you feel uncomfortable about any information being discussed, please let your nurse know and other arrangements will be made at that time. If you are sleeping at change of shift report, a nurse will "check" on you but the verbal report will be done elsewhere to permit your continued rest, unless you have asked us to wake you up for report.*
>
> *We know that Bedside Report will benefit you, the patient, by keeping you better informed of your condition. It also allows us to continue to maintain the high quality of care that you expect as a patient at (name) Hospital.*
>
> *Name, CNO*

To download a full-size version of this sample, go to the *Excellence in the Emergency Department* resource page at www.studergroup.com/excellenceintheED.

During your last hourly round on the patient prior to shift change, say, "We will be changing shifts and doing bedside report very soon. Is there anything I can get you while I am here? We will be discussing your current status and updating you on your plan of care. We want to maintain your privacy. If you have family or friends in the room with you, we'll ask you if you'd like them to step out."

2. **Use the SBAR communication technique** (Situation-Background-Assessment-Recommendation). It provides a framework for communication between members of your healthcare team. SBAR is an easy-to-remember and concrete mechanism useful for framing any conversation, including those held in front of the patient. This technique facilitates

an easy, focused way to set expectations and relay important information. (See sample.)

Figure 6.2

How to Use SBAR(T) in ED Bedside Shift Report

S = situation   B = background   A = assessment   R = recommendation   T= thank you

S	**Offgoing Nurse-** • Manage Up-–"I'm going home now. Samantha will be your nurse for the next shift. I've worked with Samantha for five years and I can tell you I'm leaving you in good hands. I always hear such nice things about her from her patients." **Oncoming Nurse-** • Introduce self using AIDET (Acknowledge, Introduce, Duration, Explanation, Thank You) • Update white board • Check armband while asking patient to state his/her name and date of birth
B	**Offgoing Nurse-** • Involve patient in change of shift report—"I'm about to give report to Samantha. Please listen so at the end you can ask any questions or fill in any additional information that Samantha will need to know to care for you during her shift. " • Give a brief update on patient's chief complaint and what treatments/medications have been provided • Update on any pending tests or treatments (i.e. lab/radiology) • Discuss any special needs (i.e. altered mental status, fall risk, isolation precautions) **Oncoming Nurse-** • Ask patient if they have any questions
A	**Offgoing Nurse-** • Give explanation—"We are going to do a quick physical assessment together since we are changing shifts." • Inform the oncoming nurse of what you have assessed and or noted during your shift • Include any information or tasks that you have completed • Mention what the oncoming nurse will need to complete or follow-up on **Oncoming Nurse-** • Review chart/check documentation • Conduct a quick physical assessment and check all IV sites/pumps for accuracy • Assess patient's pain using a pain scale
R	**Offgoing Nurse-** • Review all orders and plan of care with oncoming nurse (tests, treatments, medication therapy, IV sites/meds) • Include relevant medications that have been ordered and any ancillary or support services that are working with the patient such as respiratory therapy, radiology, social services, etc. • Ask the patient- "Do you have any questions? Is there anything else the nurse needs to know at this time?" **Oncoming Nurse-** • Validate orders/plan of care • Ask any questions of offgoing nurse
T	**Thank the Patient-** **Offgoing and Oncoming Nurse-** Prior to leaving the room, asks the patient the following: • Is your **pain** under control? • Do you understand the **plan of care**? • Do you know what you are waiting for and what will happen next? • Do you have any **concerns** we can address? **Use Closing Key Words-** • **Offgoing Nurse-** "Samantha will take very good care of you. Thank you for allowing me to care for you today." • **Oncoming Nurse-** "Is there anything you need right now? I'll be back to check on you in about an hour."

To download a full-size version of this sample format and/or a competency checklist, go to the *Excellence in the Emergency Department* resource page at www.studergroup.com/excellenceintheED.

Use a Mini-Bedside Report to Improve ED-to-Inpatient Hand-offs and Transfers

You can improve patient satisfaction and teamwork between ED and inpatient staff by using a mini-bedside report during the patient transfer. Inpatient staff should greet the patient upon arrival using AIDET (See Chapter 7) and receive a mini-bedside report from ED staff.

ED staff can say goodbye to the patient and manage up inpatient staff using key words (e.g., "Theresa will take 'very good' care of you. In fact, staff will be rounding on you hourly to ensure you receive 'excellent' care."). (Use survey words.)

Just as other bedside reports reduce errors and increase patient involvement, so too will a mini-bedside report. These also reduce the number of patients who leave against medical advice (AMA).

Tips for Success:

- **Be sensitive to privacy and information shared in front of the patient.** Use key words to let the patient know you will maintain their privacy and keep their information safe. Discuss sensitive information away from the patient's bedside to maintain confidentiality. Also, be sensitive to what you say in front of a patient. Although we may feel the patient is non-compliant, say, "The physician recommended...but the patient declined," instead of describing him or her as uncooperative.

- **Educate the oncoming nursing team** about bedside shift report if they are float or registry personnel.

- **Exclude opinions.** Report is a time for facts. If a nurse is unhappy with the patient (or physician caring for the patient), the bedside report is **not** the time to vent. Criticism makes the nurse appear less credible.

- **Avoid putting a nurse on the spot in front of the patient and/or family.** If the oncoming nurse has a question or needs clarification about a sensitive issue, wait until after bedside shift report is complete. Then ask the offgoing nurse after both nurses have left the room.

Track and Follow-up

Just as we recommend when implementing other processes (e.g., rounding for outcomes, AIDET, hourly rounding), you'll want to formalize training of staff on bedside shift report and ask an evaluator to complete a competency assessment to ensure standardization and compliance. (You can download a copy at www.studergroup.com/excellenceintheED.) Then report back wins and opportunities regularly to staff at huddles and stand-up meetings using results from the bedside report dashboard. (See sample.)

Figure 6.3

ED Bedside Weekly Report

	n size	Nurse took time to listen	Nurses informative re: treatments	Informed about delays	Staff cared about you as a person	How well pain was controlled
Baseline		50%	58%	28%	45%	58%
Goal- In Percentile Rank		50%	50%	50%	50%	50%
Week of:						
7/29 - 8/4	13	51%	76%	93%	90%	97%
8/5 - 8/11	11	87%	57%	58%	66%	8%
8/12 - 8/18	11	71%	81%	19%	21%	50%
8/19 - 8/25	11	87%	87%	6%	72%	67%
8/26 - 9/1	8	14%	81%	25%	26%	75%
9/2 - 9/8	11	93%	93%	78%	88%	91%
9/9 - 9/15	1	72%	61%	69%	81%	64%
9/16 - 9/22	1	62%	99%	99%	99%	81%
9/23 - 9/29	3	90%	99%	99%	99%	99%
9/30 - 10/6	7	76%	80%	92%	82%	76%
10/7 - 10/13	1	99%	99%	91%	99%	99%

Baseline= May - July
Report = Pt response by Date of Discharge. Note: Weekly results may change over time

To download a full-size blank version of this template, go to the *Excellence in the Emergency Department* resource page at www. studergroup.com/excellenceintheED.

In closing...

Will patients notice when you implement bedside shift report? Read this patient story submitted by CNO Connie Huber at Providence St. Peter Hospital in Olympia, WA, during their pilot of bedside shift report. Providence St. Peter uses bedside reports in all units, including ED, to reduce patient anxiety and build trust and confidence.

"My Confidence in My Care Grew Exponentially"

Due to cardiology issues, I have been hospitalized for seven lengthy stays in the past 13 months, at three different hospitals. My greatest care concern, besides the bills and getting better, was the dreaded shift change. With so many different nurse personalities, I was often left wondering if my nurses truly understood my condition, meds, or progress.

Were they actually even in communication with my doctor?

Then came the fear of starting over again with a new nurse just 12 hours later (or sooner)! I often wondered what was being said behind my back or if there was even time to update my new nurse with an accurate report. The fear of the unknown felt like a weapon formed against me.

To my delight and surprise, Providence St. Peter Hospital changed all that for me two days ago when my night nurse personally introduced me to my day nurse and then proceeded to systematically recall my case, symptoms, and medications with a full bedside report.

I couldn't believe my ears! My own concerns were actually heard by both nurses and I had the opportunity to interject and clarify.

A new confidence in my care grew exponentially in that short 10 minutes! I thought it would be extinguished when the next shift came on but once again I was introduced and then included in the bedside report. What an exciting relief.

Thank you, St. Peter staff, for stepping up to this healthy level of patient care communication. You are now my *only* hospital!

—A Grateful Patient

Key Learning Points: Bedside Shift Report

1. Bedside shift report offers real-time information exchange between the oncoming and offgoing nurses and patient at the patient's bedside.

2. It's a critical patient safety tactic to prevent medical errors during shift changes and also builds employee teamwork, ownership, trust, and accountability.

3. In the ED, bedside shift report takes two to three minutes. Before entering the patient's room, the oncoming nurse will review the patient's chart, history, and treatments. Then the two nurses go together to the bedside, introduce themselves using AIDET, and report using the SBAR communication technique and involving the patient.

4. Use key words to let the patient know his privacy is your top concern. Ask the patient if he would like family or friends to leave during bedside shift report. Also, sensitive information can be communicated between nurses away from the bedside as appropriate.

5. Bedside shift report should be implemented only after hard wiring leader rounding on staff and leader rounding on patients.

6. Train, track, and follow-up. You'll want to formally train staff on bedside report using a competency assessment to ensure compliance and standardization. Use the Bedside Report Dashboard to report back wins and opportunities to staff at huddles and stand-up meetings.

Advanced Tactics to Accelerate and Sustain Success

CHAPTER 7

Key Words at Key Times

*"Ten percent is what life brings you. Ninety percent is
what you do and say."*
— Alice Crowe

What Are Key Words?

Key words are not new. We use them each day when we say,
"Excuse me," "Please," or "Thank you." Key words are a verbal
signal that links an action to a behavior to create a common understanding.

It's not about patient satisfaction or "smile school." It's about
being prescriptive and consistent in the ED. It's about reducing patient anxiety and ensuring that we are providing safe care...which
is what we signed up for.

In the ED, some key words—like "Stat!" and "Code Blue"—
stimulate an immediate response. We access resources right away
to save a patient's life. We say, "Stand clear!" as a safety precaution
for our employees when we defibrillate a patient.

And yet, while key words are commonly used, they are not
always commonly practiced. When they *are* used consistently, they
provide a powerful way to communicate our intentions. When we
say, "I am closing the curtain for your privacy," for example, the

patients don't wonder if we're closing the curtain as a way to avoid them.

We also use key words to be compliant with the Emergency Medical Treatment and Active Labor Act (EMTALA) regulations, which mandate that ED staff do not use words that encourage patients to leave without treatment. Using verbiage such as, "You can wait, but it will be at least eight hours," or, "You may want to try XYZ ED down the street," is not appropriate.

Rather, your goal is to use verbiage that does not encourage patients to leave. You want to reassure them that it's safe to wait. You can say, "There is a wait right now, but per your assessment, we feel comfortable that it's safe for you to wait. We'll be back to check on you within the hour. If you feel your condition is worsening, please let us know."

Another benefit: When non-clinical staff are rounding on patients in the ED, key words ensure consistency in our communications. (However, clinical issues should always be referred to the triage nurse.)

In Studer Group's experience, some of the very most effective key words are "AIDET"SM (Acknowledge–Introduce–Duration–Explanation–Thank You), which I'll introduce in this chapter. We call them the Five Fundamentals of Service because of their proven ability to reduce patient anxiety, increase patient compliance, improve outcomes, and manage patient expectations.

How Many Key Words Do We Need?

Use key words to address pain, plan of care, and to keep patients informed in the ED. Use them for any behavior that you want the staff to do consistently. Studer Group also recommends you choose key words based on patient priorities. Get staff buy-in by letting them be part of the process in choosing three or four sets of key words that support patient safety or the patient experience. Then be relentless about using them.

What often happens is that leaders try to introduce too many key words and the staff rebel. Instead, prioritize around the priority questions on your survey (e.g., pain, plan of care, and duration). Also, choose key words that are associated with safety, such as: "I am going to ask you your name and date of birth and check your armband to keep you safe." This helps patients recognize your organization's commitment to safety.

Sometimes leaders will say to me, "We tried key words, but they didn't really make a difference. They just didn't work for us." Why might this be? First of all, to have an impact, you need to be using them frequently enough for patients to notice. Secondly, remember that staff will use key words consistently only if there are just a few sets of key words you ask them to use. Remember that less is more. To achieve results, hold staff accountable for the key words your team chooses to use.

In one ED that I worked in, we noticed that patients routinely left their clothing on the chair, leaving nowhere for family members or the physician to sit. Since having physicians sit with patients was a high priority for us, we put hooks on the wall and used the key words, "For your convenience, please hang your clothes on the hook so your physician or family member can sit in the chair when they come in."

Key words are used in many industries outside of healthcare. Once when I was presenting on key words, I asked my audience if they'd ever worked at a fast food restaurant when they were younger. Many said yes.

"How long would you keep your job at McDonald's if you showed up without your uniform and name tag?" I asked them. "Or what if you were working the drive-thru and were supposed to say, 'Would you like to try the special today?' but you opted out?"

One guy actually answered me. He said, "An hour. I got fired because I didn't use the key words in the drive-thru!"

And just think...you probably wouldn't die if you, as a McDonald's customer, got the wrong order because the drive-thru guy forgot his key words. But your patients could die in the ED if you forget key words. What if you give a patient the wrong medication because you forget to say, "Mrs. Jones, can you please state your full name and date of birth while I check your armband for safety?"

Key Words: The Good, the Bad, and the Ugly

Over the years, because we have the opportunity to travel the country so frequently, Studer Group's ED coaches have come across a fair number of interesting key words and signage in the ED.

I'm sure you'd never use any of the "Top 10 Worst Key Words" in your ED, but we have surely heard them! To improve your patients' experience, work with your staff to adopt the "Better Key Words" for every patient, every time.

Figure 7.1

Top 10 Key Words and Better Key Words

Top 10 Worst Key Words	Better Key Words
1. Why are you here for this?	1. How can I help you today?
2. I have no idea how long it will take.	2. Your labs should take about an hour to come back. If it is longer, I will be back to update you.
3. You can't go back right now.	3. Let me check and see when you can see your son.
4. The physician is really busy right now.	4. The doctor is with another patient right now, but should be in to see you in the next 15 minutes.
5. You need to stay in your room.	5. Let me update you on why you are waiting. Is there anything you need right now?
6. No, you can't have anything to eat or drink right now.	6. I know you must be hungry and thirsty. Let me explain why the physician doesn't want you to eat or drink right now.
7. I'm not your nurse.	7. Sarah is your nurse. Let me ask her to come in and answer your questions.
8. I'd love to discharge you, but we are still waiting on the lab to give us your results. They are always slow this time of day.	8. We are waiting for one more lab test to come back. This will take about another 20 minutes and then the physician can review all of your results with you.
9. You should be able to go to radiology "in just a little bit."	9. You should be able to go to radiology in the next 20 minutes.
10. We are short-staffed and can't go any faster!	10. I apologize you had to wait. Is there anything you need right now?

To download a full-size version of this sample, go to the *Excellence in the Emergency Department* resource page at www.studergroup.com/excellenceintheED.

We have also seen some pretty interesting signs in Emergency Departments. There was the one that read: "Please be advised that Registration has no control over wait times. If your condition worsens, please see the triage nurse."

Another read: "Please don't leave! If you are not here when your name is called, your chart will be put at the back of the line and your waiting time will start over. Thanks for your cooperation."

You know, it's easy for us to get too close to what we see every day. We can walk right by that light that's been out for a week, a curtain that's dirty, or signs like those above. My suggestion: Ask someone who doesn't work in the department to walk it with you with fresh eyes from the patient perspective. Is there anything that doesn't make a great impression on patients? Fix it. Are signs welcoming and informative? Does staff explain why we do what we do? Are there any changes you can make to improve the patient experience while they wait?

Sample Key Words to Use for Rounding in the ED Reception Area

When you round hourly in the ED reception area, the goal is to show care and compassion to patients and families and to reassure them that they are safe to wait. (See Chapter 4 to learn more about rounding in the reception area.) Remember, they are feeling anxious about their emergency. Let them know you will keep them informed and check on them hourly. Tell them what to do if their condition worsens.

An example:

"Hello. I'm Suzanne, the triage nurse. I know I saw you a couple of hours ago. I apologize for the wait. I want to make sure you're okay. Let me take a look at your laceration. That's great that the bandage looks dry. A bed should be available in the next 30 minutes. Now, if you start to bleed through that bandage, I want you to come and see me."

Figure 7.2

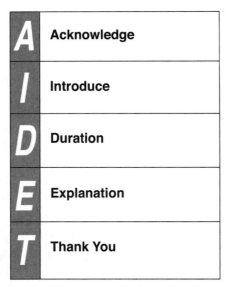

AIDET:
The Five Fundamentals of Service

"AIDET" is just an acronym for the Five Fundamentals of Service.

These are:

A	**Acknowledge**
I	**Introduce**
D	**Duration**
E	**Explanation**
T	**Thank You**

A *stands for Acknowledge.* Acknowledgment is the first opportunity to make a person real. Studer Group recommends the "10-5" rule with respect to acknowledgment. In other words, at 10 feet, look up, smile, and make eye contact to demonstrate approach-ability. At 5 feet, acknowledge them verbally (e.g., "Good morning. How are you?").

Also, use the patient's last name if possible. In their article "An Evidence-Based Perspective on Greetings in Medical Encounters,"[1] the authors write, "Because greetings are one way to ensure proper identification of patients, they may well be considered a fundamental component of patient safety." In fact, 91.3 percent of patients wanted to be addressed by their name.[2]

So, in summary: Make eye contact. Make the patient feel that you expected them. Acknowledge the individual to let the patient know that you know they are there.

I know it's not easy. When I was a new grad who was just struggling to manage all my patients, I made particularly good eye contact with the IV bag and the chart. I'd go into the patient's room, look at all the monitors and check that the side rails were up...I was very task-oriented. But I didn't spend much time getting to eye level with the patient or acknowledging them. Since those days, I've learned that the person is much more important than the task.

I *stands for Introduce.* Tell the patient your name, title, and credentials so she knows who will be caring for her. At Studer Group, this is considered "first generation I."

I know some of your ED staff may be reluctant to introduce themselves in the beginning. In the old days, some staff may have been told not to give out their name in the ED. You could be stalked by a drug seeker or angry patient, right? But you know what? That's unlikely. And in today's world, transparency reigns. The Patient Bill of Rights says that at all times patients must know who is caring for them and in what role.

It's also our responsibility. We have to put the patient first. So if you need to help your staff become more comfortable introducing themselves, ask them: "What part of this is not right for the patient?" We introduce ourselves not for our comfort, but for the comfort of the patient

"Next generation I" also includes an introduction that "manages up"—or positions positively—yourself, your skill set, experience, and certifications, as well as coworkers and other departments. You might say, "Hello, Mrs. Williams, my name is Jim Johnson. I'm the Emergency Department technician and I'll be helping to care for you today. Here at Memorial, patient satisfaction is very important to us so I want to be sure you receive excellent care. I've been in healthcare for 20 years now...the last five years right here at Memorial ED. You're very fortunate that Dr. Campbell is your emergency physician today. She is one of our very best."

Sometimes staff push back on managing up their skill set and experience. "We're not going to do that," they'll say. "It sounds like we're bragging." Here's a tip to help staff get past the uncomfortable barrier. When you greet the patient, after introducing yourself, ask the patient: "Is this your first time here?" Whether the patient says yes or no, his answer provides an opening to manage up staff skill set and experience.

If the patient says yes, the staff can say, "We're glad you're here. We have a great team to care for you." If the patient says no, they can say, "Welcome back! I've worked here 10 years and I love it. I just want you to know that you're in great hands." Then it doesn't sound phony or fake.

When speaking to staff about the need to manage up experience, take it back to the patient as you did with the introduction. What's not right about the patient knowing a little bit about the people taking care of him? It reduces patient anxiety and builds trust and credibility.

D *stands for Duration.* How long will the wait/test/procedure/visit take? How long until the results are available? How long before the doctor comes in? ED folks always tell me, "But I don't know how long it's going to be!" So should we just let them wait for six hours and hope they don't notice?

No, we can't be afraid of what I call "the big bad D" (duration).

Here's the thing: Time is either real or perceived. Have you ever heard a patient say, "I've been here three hours and no one has told me anything?!" And then, when you look at the chart, you see the patient has actually waited only an hour and a half?

In my experience as a nurse manager, patients who complain about wait times (because they have not been given an expectation for wait time) will enhance the time they waited from 25 to 50 percent!

In one 2009 patient satisfaction study of nearly 1.4 million patients treated at 1,725 EDs nationwide, **patients who reported they received "good" or "very good" information about delays reported nearly the same satisfaction, whether they had spent over four hours or less than one hour in the ED.**[3] So the good news is, you can still achieve high patient satisfaction when your patients have to wait, as long as you make the time to keep patients informed.

We have to tell them something. And you know what? We know. We know that if a patient comes in with abdominal pain, they're likely going to spend the next four hours with us. If they're getting fluids and pain meds and they have to get a CT of the abdomen with contrast, then we'll need to see how they do and if they can tolerate liquids before they go home. They're going to be here for the afternoon. So tell them. Under-promise, then over-deliver. Patients will give us lots of latitude if we are honest in our communications with them.

When possible, offer concrete time expectations. If that time passes, don't worry that you didn't make the goal. Just return to the patient and update them.

Some EDs have identified agreed upon times for common tests. They say, "We know your labs will take 45 minutes to an hour. If it's going to be longer, we'll let you know."

Other EDs have even produced signage that defines average time frames for routine diagnostic procedures such as labs and x-rays. Signage can be a good thing, as long as we manage expectations to the times we give the patient. When you approach a waiting room door with an angry patient or family behind it, chances are good that the anger will be directly proportionate to the amount of information they have been given or not given. That's why we use key words for "informed about delays" when we round on patients in the reception area.

E *stands for Explanation.* The explanation is the quality piece... the important part, because it connects back to clinical quality and patient safety. In one study, two of the top four factors that engendered complete trust in a physician were: 1) the patient got as much medical information as they wanted; and 2) the patient was told what to do if symptoms continued, worsened, or returned.[4]

When a patient leaves your ED, it's important that they have a very clear understanding about what you want them to do once they are home. In fact, in studies of patient behavior[5], only half the patients who leave a doctor's office will take the medication. According to the Office of the Inspector General, noncompliance with medications results in 125,000 deaths each year from cardiovascular disease alone.

In the ED, we have three opportunities to explain or use key words to ensure patients are compliant with our care at the end of their visit. First, when a physician does a formal close with a patient, he or she is essentially contracting with the patient that they will be compliant with discharge instructions.

Secondly, nurses can manage up physicians and reinforce expectations by saying, "I know Dr. Smith has shared with you the discharge instructions. What questions do you still have?" Offer information about what will happen next and what the patient should expect. Ask: "Do you understand your discharge instructions?"

In fact, I recommend you "over-explain." This ensures your patients are hearing what you say. After providing discharge instructions, say: "Tell me what you heard. What more information do you need on that?"

And thirdly, the last opportunity to ensure patients are compliant with discharge instructions is during the discharge phone call. An excellent time to check in is within 72 hours after the patient goes home to learn if prescriptions were filled, if the patient needs further instructions, and to see how he or she is doing. You will put the patient at ease by letting them know that you anticipated they might have additional questions and that you have the time and interest to answer them.

T *stands for Thank You.* Your patients have a choice and if they don't have a positive experience and there's a wait, maybe they'll just drive right past you to the ED down the street. So say, "Thanks for coming in today," or, "Thanks for letting me take care of you," or, "Thanks for choosing General Hospital. Is there anything else you need before you go? Any other questions I can answer?"

This is not about saying, "Thank you for shopping at K-mart." The point is to show care and compassion for patients and their families who may be dealing with difficult situations when the patient goes home.

A thank you also allows an opening for the patient to thank your staff for the care they have given them and to have a final moment to say goodbye. In my experience, patients often take this extra moment to share their appreciation for the care they have received.

The Power of AIDET

AIDET is an evidence-based leadership practice. In Studer Group's experience, organizations that use it relentlessly get impressive results.

An example: Parkwest Medical Center (a member of Covenant Health) in Knoxville, TN, has been above the 90th percentile in patient satisfaction for the last three years. They credit their success to their implementation of AIDET, key words, discharge phone calls, and hourly rounds (which we cover in Chapter 8).

In fact, Diana Shaffer, nurse manager at Parkwest Emergency Care Center says, "The outcomes were produced by a relentless focus on employee and physician engagement and patient-centered care. Our three years of outstanding results are proof that these strategies work. Just do it!"

When we use AIDET, patients are less anxious and more compliant with their plan of care. AIDET also responds directly to National Patient Safety Goal #13: "Encourage patients' active involvement in their own care as a patient safety strategy." AIDET includes talking directly to patients about their plan of care and asking them if they can commit to it. This drives better clinical outcomes.

And the icing on the cake? Patients feel good about their experience, which increases patient satisfaction.

In fact, I tell people that **AIDET and key words combined with leader rounding on patients will address every single complaint I've ever heard!** AIDET is common sense, but not always commonly practiced. For it to work, we need to use it, as appropriate, during every patient encounter.

Figure 7.3

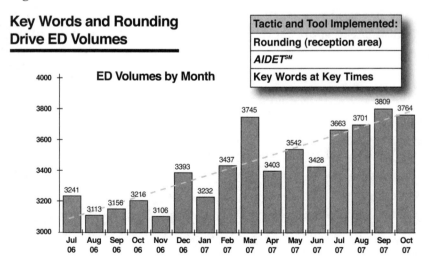

Key Words and Rounding Drive ED Volumes

| Tactic and Tool Implemented: |
| Rounding (reception area) |
| *AIDET*^{SM} |
| Key Words at Key Times |

Source: Texas Hospital, Admissions: 12,705, ED Visits: 40,000, Employees: 1,611

This Texas hospital credits its steady increase in monthly volumes to rounding in the ED reception area and use of AIDET and Key Words at Key Times.

Just a few months ago, I was teaching AIDET and a leader at one of the hospitals I coach came up to me and said, "I really didn't believe you about the power of AIDET until just this last week."

"What happened this week?" I asked her.

She said, "Well, I was on my way home from Italy, and there was a whole lot of turbulence on the airplane. I got scared…white knuckles and the whole thing.

"And then the pilot came on the loudspeaker. 'I've been flying this plane for 25 years,' he said. 'And I've had a lot of experience with this kind of turbulence, so I want to put you at ease.'

"I felt so much better after he said that," she said. "I might just use AIDET after all."

Using AIDET to Manage Up Others

"Managing up" refers to putting others in a positive light. If you're my patient and are leaving to go to Radiology, I can say, "Well, good luck over there. I'll see you back in a couple of hours because they're always short-staffed this time of day…but it doesn't matter because we've got patients waiting to go upstairs anyway, so you're not going anywhere soon."

Or I can say, "You are in luck today. Paul is going to do your chest x-ray. He is excellent and will take great care of you."

We have multiple opportunities every day in the ED to manage up, to manage neutral, or to manage down. When we choose to manage up, we really do reduce patients' anxiety and increase their willingness to do the things we are asking them to do. But it's our choice. And it's a choice we must make actively every time.

As a leader, you can manage up your staff by:

- giving praise at the bedside
- always expecting excellence

- mentoring ceaselessly
- holding people accountable for poor behavior

At the last ED I managed before I became a coach for Studer Group, we were barely cracking the 4th percentile in patient satisfaction. Nowhere to go but up. I knew it would be critical to role model and practice what I preached.

But it wasn't easy. I had to actively work at it every single day…giving praise to my staff in front of the patients. I'd say, "I see that Pauline is your nurse today. You're in good hands. You have one of the best nurses that we have." That shared confidence leverages trust for the patient and your staff. As a result of our success with AIDET, rounding in the reception area, bedside report, and discharge phone calls, we moved patient satisfaction to the 98th percentile in just over 14 months!

But What If I Don't Have Anything Nice to Say?

A suggestion: When you're feeling frustrated or emotional and you just don't have anything nice to say, go back to the objective data. You can still say, "Unfortunately, Radiology is running late today. It will be another 30 minutes. However, I know that once you get in there, they are going to take very good care of you."

Or you could really manage up staff in the department. You could say, "Roberta is working in the Radiology Department today. She's going to take great care of you, keep you informed, and you'll be back here in less than 15 minutes."

When I was a nurse manager, I had an ED physician who was very thorough but very slow. I used to say to him, "What am I going to tell my patients about you? I love you to death but you're killing me here! You've got to get moving so we can see all these patients!"

Finally, we made a deal. And here's how I managed him up to patients. I'd say, "Mr. James, Dr. Thompson is going to come in to see you. You're really lucky today that Dr. Thompson is going to be your physician. It is going to be another 20 minutes because he is spending time with another patient right now. But I assure you that when he comes in, he will spend time with you, let you know what's going to happen next, and answer all your questions."

It's all about being honest and managing up strengths.

How Do You Know If Staff Are Using Key Words and AIDET Every Time?

First, observe some patient interactions. You may hear only a snippet of an acknowledgment and introduction in triage or overhear someone's discharge instructions as you pass a treatment room, but you will learn if staff are using key words and AIDET. Ask the management team to each listen for 10 direct observations per month when you get started.

The goal is to observe the staff and look for evidence that they are using AIDET. If a nurse manager walks by a patient treatment room and hears a nurse say, "Now remember, Mr. Pratt, it's going to be about 45 minutes until your labs come back," he has just heard evidence of duration.

After observing the interaction, give feedback to the staff in the spirit of collaboration and learning. Tell them the things they did really well and where they had opportunity for improvement. Leader rounding on patients is an important way that leaders can verify that staff are using AIDET when they round on patients.

Also, monitor your patient satisfaction survey results. Are responses to the question about courtesy improving as staff introduce themselves more consistently? Look at the verbatim patient comments to find evidence.

You'll know your staff are using AIDET when you read comments like, "I really enjoyed having Janette as my nurse. She explained my plan of care." Or: "My nurse told me she has worked here for 20 years." "She told me how long everything would take."

Sometimes patients literally write out AIDET in their comments. Take a look at the excerpt from this letter to the editor that was sent by a grateful mother about her experience at Fort Sanders Sevier Medical Center in Sevierville, TN:

Dear Editor,

On May 4, I accompanied my 19-year-old son to the Emergency Room at Fort Sanders Sevier County Hospital. I would like to take a moment to publicly thank the folks that took care of us that day. The woman at the front desk, **Sonya, our triage nurse, Greg, our nurses Megan and Wendy, the lab tech, Kimberly, and Dr. Kochert** were all kind, capable, and caring. It was an exceptional experience. They were quite **professional and comforting** in this stressful time of illness.

There was a television in our room to help with the wait and if it was taking extra time **someone came to explain the situation to us. It helped to ease a lot of our anxiety to have each person we came in contact with explain everything to us. We felt involved, proactive, and cared for.**

When my son needed **fast and efficient medical care, he not only got that but we met some of the kindest people we have encountered**. I believe that we are very fortunate to have them.

Sincerely,
Ronda K. Cruise

It's so important to transfer these tactics beyond the ED to other departments as well, to ensure a positive patient experience across the organization. Here's another letter from a patient at Parkwest Comprehensive Breast Center in Knoxville, TN:

> Today I had my first mammogram. From the moment I walked through the door at Parkwest, I knew I was going to have a great experience. Deborah and Melanie at the front desk were very accommodating as they helped me fill out all the forms. Next, I was greeted by nurse Bonnie. She gave me step-by-step directions that eased my anxiety. She was extremely professional and was great at her job. Before I could blink an eye, the procedure was over!
>
> Thanks to Bonnie, all those terrible stories about pain and discomfort did not apply to me. When I mentioned that I would be leaving town within two days, and was afraid I would miss the call to hear my results, sweet Bonnie called me on my cell phone shortly after I left the procedure to tell me the good news!
>
> Again, I would like to commend this group on their ability to make a woman feel comfortable during a very necessary test. You ladies rock!
>
> Sincerely,
> Barbara Elkins

It's also important to add a little fun when implementing new practices! When I started AIDET in my ED, I ran a fun little contest where I held a prize drawing for the first person to get their name mentioned five times in the patient survey comment section. I knew if they were getting mentioned, they were introducing themselves. As we got better, we had to move to a quarterly drawing because so many people were being named! The more we rewarded and recognized, the more evidence there was that staff were using AIDET.

Effective communication is a vital part of providing excellent care. AIDET and key words bring consistency, reduce anxiety, increase compliance, reduce errors, and improve the overall patient experience. They make all the difference between treating a patient like a number or as a real person who is experiencing what they consider to be an emergent event in their life...one that they may remember us by forever!

Key Learning Points: Key Words at Key Times

1. We use Key Words at Key Times in the ED so patients know why we are doing what we are doing, to be compliant with EMTALA regulations, and to ensure consistency in our communications to reduce patient anxiety and increase safety.

2. Use key words for pain, plan of care, and keeping patients informed (duration) since these match patient priorities in the ED. Choose a few key words and key times and then use them with every patient every time. Be relentless!

3. Key words are used to keep patients informed about delays when rounding in the ED reception area.

4. "AIDET" stands for Acknowledge-Introduce-Duration-Explanation-Thank You. These are the Five Fundamentals of Service. They reduce patient anxiety, increase patient compliance with the plan of care, and improve clinical outcomes.

5. You can use AIDET to "manage up"—portray in a positive light—yourself, your experience, your skill set, and those of physicians and other departments. This practice creates seamless hand-offs and transfers the trust you have built with a patient to your coworker for better outcomes.

6. Managing up is not "bragging." It's an evidence-based leadership practice in the best interest of patients. Likewise, you can always find something truthful and helpful to say about a colleague…even if you have to be creative!

CHAPTER 8

Hourly Rounding with Individualized Patient Care in the ED

"Build good habits. Habit one—Be proactive."
—Franklin Covey

When a woman died in the ED lobby of a Los Angeles hospital recently, it made national news. The woman's husband had called 911 and asked the dispatcher to send an ambulance to take them to another hospital because his wife was vomiting blood and not getting any help.

"Why aren't they helping her in the emergency room where you already are?" the dispatcher asked.

"They're just watching her and they're not doing anything," he answered.

On that day, Americans around the country wondered how this could happen in U.S. healthcare today. They wondered if it could happen to them.

But consider this: If every ED in the country implemented hourly rounding in their treatment and reception areas, this kind of event would be highly unlikely to reoccur. **Hourly rounding in the ED is another evidence-based leadership practice that keeps patients safe and ensures they receive timely, appropriate care.** Hourly rounding with individualized patient care is even more effective because it ensures staff are responding to what is most important to each patient.

About the ED Hourly Rounding Study

Many of you may be familiar with the 2006 Studer Alliance for Health Care Research study, which revealed that rounding every one to two hours on hospital inpatient units significantly reduced patients' use of call lights, reduced falls, and improved patient satisfaction.[1]

Since 51 percent of inpatients come from the Emergency Department and typically judge their inpatient experience based on their ED experience, it was a logical next step to test the power of hourly rounding in the ED. And so, in late 2006, based on significant interest expressed by nurses, the Studer Alliance for Health Care Research launched an ED study, which was published on-line in the *Journal of Emergency Medicine*. You can read the complete study results at www.studergroup.com/excellenceintheED.

Thirty-two EDs participated in the six-week study (71 percent were Studer Group partners while 29 percent were not). All participants were required to have implemented leader rounding on staff and patients as a prerequisite to inclusion in the study.

In addition to hourly rounding, Studer Group decided to include the individualized patient care tactic that was also proving to be very successful on inpatient units.

As a result, three different rounding treatments were tested during the study:

1. Hourly rounding in triage and reception areas
2. Hourly rounding with individualized patient care in triage and reception areas (Individualized patient care—responding to the most important priority of each patient—was accomplished by using whiteboards, cards, or stickers.)

3. Rounding every 30 minutes in the triage and reception areas was assigned to any ED with a treat and release time of under 150 minutes

The Hypotheses

Based on results from the inpatient call light study, we believed that hourly rounding in the ED would: increase patient satisfaction; reduce patients who left without being seen (LWOBS); reduce patients leaving against medical advice (AMA); reduce call lights; reduce families and patients approaching the nursing station; reduce patient falls; increase awareness of ED staff behaviors; and impact MDs to improve their behaviors.

The Eight Behaviors Tested

Participating EDs rounded every 30 minutes or hourly and:

1. Used opening key words or actions to introduce themselves, their skill set, and experience;
2. Performed scheduled tasks (e.g., giving physician-ordered medication, starting an IV, wound care);
3. Addressed pain, plan of care, and duration (wait times);
4. Assessed additional comfort needs (e.g., warm blanket, pillow, ice);
5. Conducted an environmental assessment (e.g., call light within reach, warm blanket, side rails up);
6. Used closing key words and/or actions;
7. Explained when they or someone else would return; and
8. Documented the round on the log or chart.

Why did we choose these eight behaviors?

Because they respond to those top three priorities of all ED patients that we discussed earlier: PPD...or pain, plan of care, and duration. ED patients want to have their pain controlled; want staff and physicians to keep them informed about their plan of care; and want to be kept informed about delays. These hourly rounding behaviors also directly respond to National Patient Safety Goal 13: "Encourage patients' active involvement in their own care as a patient safety strategy."

The Study Results

- **Fewer patients left without being seen. There was a decrease of 23.4 percent LWOBS overall among all participating EDs.** The 30-minute rounding group saw a 19.7 percent reduction; the one-hour rounding group saw an 18.5 percent reduction; and hourly rounding with IPC saw a 33.2 percent reduction. Consider the combined financial impact on these 32 EDs that kept an additional 463 patients. At $500 net revenue per patient, they earned $231,500 during the six-week rounding experiment.

- **Fewer patients who left against medical advice (AMA). There was an overall decrease of 22.6 percent AMA in participating EDs.** The 30-minute rounding group saw a 24.1 percent reduction; the one-hour rounding group saw a 17 percent reduction; and hourly rounding with IPC saw a 37.1 percent reduction. Financial impact: Capturing $200 net revenue[2] per patient on 162 patients created a $32,400 cost savings.

- **Fewer patient falls. There was an overall decrease of 58.8 percent in falls.** The hourly rounding group saw a 54.5 percent reduction while the group doing hourly rounding with individualized patient care saw a 66.7 percent reduction. Financial impact: Ten fewer falls at a cost of $11,042 per patient created a savings of $110,420. This positive financial impact is particularly important since the Center for Medicare and Medicaid Services (CMS) has designated patient falls as a Serious Preventable Adverse Event (SPAE). CMS no longer reimburses for them.

- **Fewer patients using call lights. There was a 34.7 percent reduction overall in call light usage.** If we use an estimate of four minutes to get to the room, fulfill the patient's need or request and return to the task the nurse was doing before being interrupted—a time estimate that most nurses would find low—nurses in the study gained 584 hours that they could redirect to other patient care tasks.

- **Fewer families and patients approaching the nursing station.** There was a 39.5 percent reduction overall in the study! This was good news as it meant these EDs were meeting the patient and family needs more consistently during the hourly rounds. Fewer interruptions gave staff more time to document and spend time with their patients.

- **Patient satisfaction increased significantly.** Hospitals using a 5-point scale saw statistically significant changes in patients' ratings of their overall ED care, their ratings of pain management, and their ratings of being kept informed about delays. On average, patient satisfaction increased from 5 to 20 mean points in each of the categories measured.

- **ED staff perceived themselves to be more effective.** When the pre- and post-survey ratings were compared on the ED nurse and tech surveys, staff perceived they were more effective at introducing themselves to patients, communicating about the plan of care, telling patients when they'd return, giving patients an estimate of the wait time, and remembering to ask if patients had questions.

- **ED physicians, including mid-level providers (e.g., NP, PA), perceived themselves to be better at communicating** with and updating patients on their plan of care as well as assisting in pain management. These results were also based on comparing the pre- and post-survey ratings. It's important to note that these providers were not actively involved in the rounding study; however, these findings show how staff behaviors positively influenced their behavior.

Overall, the study results clearly showed that hourly rounding with individualized patient care was at least 33 percent more effective than the hourly rounding alone across almost all measures.

Why Is Individualized Patient Care So Effective?

Individualized patient care is simple. Caregivers just ask: "What is the one thing I can do for you to make sure you get very good or excellent care today?" For one patient it might be as simple as, "Make sure I can leave here by 2 p.m. so I can pick up my son from school." Another might say, "I want my husband to be with me while I wait."

Individualized patient care is a great way to begin care and to manage up staff. For example, if a patient says the most important thing we can do is manage her pain, the person rounding can say, "I'm going to let Dr. Jones know right away. We have a pain protocol so I'm also going to get you something for your pain now."

With individualized patient care, patients don't have to wait to see the physician to get some relief! We can start meeting and exceeding the patient's expectations immediately because we know what's most important to them.

The EDs that were rounding hourly with individualized patient care in the study used a card like the one below (completed at triage or when the patient was roomed and then kept with the chart) or wrote the question on the whiteboard in the treatment room to ensure that all caregivers understood the patient's top priority.

Figure 8.1

Individualized Patient Care

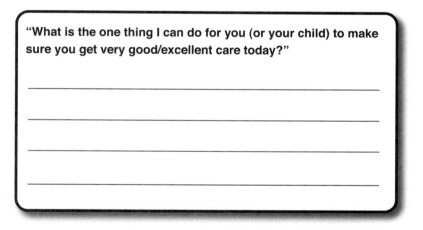

"What is the one thing I can do for you (or your child) to make sure you get very good/excellent care today?"

To download a full-size version of this sample, go to the *Excellence in the Emergency Department* resource page at www.studergroup.com/excellenceintheED.

Why We Round Hourly in the ED

Now that you've seen the data for yourself, help your staff become believers. When you begin hourly rounding in your ED, be sure to connect back to why you are doing it. To recap: Hourly rounding decreases both LWOBS and AMA rates and positively impacts patient safety, quality, and peace of mind. It saves nurses time by decreasing call lights. And it decreases falls, which results in better patient safety and higher quality care. Rounding hourly in the ED also raises patient satisfaction, which creates more loyal patients, decreases complaints, and reduces litigation.

How to Get Started

Rounding hourly in the ED is not a first tactic to use. **Be sure you have hardwired leader rounding on staff and patients as well as discharge phone calls before introducing hourly rounding on patients.** This ensures that you have strong communication with your staff and patients as well as methods to validate staff behaviors after the patient visit.

In particular, discharge phone calls offer an excellent last communication opportunity with your patient to validate whether hourly rounding occurred consistently. It's a final touch point before the patient fills out the survey. Plus, people tend to give their most honest feedback after they've left the ED.

Leader rounding on staff is a critical first process because it is the mechanism by which we give staff feedback when we implement new processes like hourly rounding. Remember, too, that hourly rounding on patients in the ED is staff-owned. You can gain that kind of ownership only by engaging employees regularly through leader rounding.

You will need to make some decisions before you begin hourly rounding. First, which tactic will you implement? We recommend implementing hourly rounding with individualized patient care due to its superior performance in the study. Then you'll need to decide who will round on patients. (See Chapter 4 for some recommendations.) And finally, you'll need to decide how to document results.

We recommend that you use a 24-hour rounding log for hourly rounding. As we recommended in Chapter 4, use the hourly rounding log in the ED reception area as well as in treatment rooms.

Figure 8.2

ED Hourly Rounding Log with
Individualized Patient Care in Treatment Area

Hospital:_____   Date:_____

Inform patient of PLAN OF CARE, inquire about PAIN and inform of any DELAYS (PPD)

TIME PERIOD	INITIALS OF PERSON ROUNDING	TIME OF ROUNDING VISIT	WRITE IN PT EXPECTATION FOR EACH PATIENT. IF A NEW PATIENT COMES INTO THE ROOM INDICATE IT WITH AN N=NEW. Note if room is empty=E
6-7 AM			
7-8 AM			
8-9 AM			
9-10 AM			
10-11 AM			
11-12 AM			
12-1 PM			
1-2 PM			
2-3 PM			
3-4 PM			
4-5 PM			
5-6 PM			
6-7 PM			
7-8 PM			
8-9 PM			
9-10 PM			
10-11 PM			
11-12 PM			
12-1 AM			
1-2 AM			
2-3 AM			
3-4 AM			
4-5 AM			
5-6 AM			

LOGS WILL BE GIVEN TO NURSE MANAGER DAILY AND REVIEWED DAILY FOR ACCOUNTABILITY.

Key= E to denote room is empty

To download a full-size version of this sample, go to the *Excellence in the Emergency Department* resource page at www.studergroup.com/excellenceintheED.

Keep the log in the treatment room as patients come and go. When rounding, if the room is empty, staff can write "room empty" or "E." That way when leaders review the log they don't think someone has forgotten to round or document the round. This validates that each assigned individual is actually rounding, so you can ensure rounding takes place consistently for 100 percent compliance.

I also suggest you create a monthly dashboard to capture results of questions from your survey (e.g., informed about delays, how well pain was controlled) and other metrics such as falls, call lights, and average turnaround time. This gives you the data to track, measure, and report back on trends, opportunities, and the financial impact of hourly rounding in the ED so everyone understands the important difference it's making in your organization.

Figure 8.3

ED Hourly Rounds Dashboard

ED	QUALITY/SAFETY			QUALITY OF LIFE FOR STAFF		PATIENT SATISFACTION								PERCENTILE RANK
	Average Turn Around Time	FALL RATE	CALL LIGHT VOL	Pts/Family approaching nurses station	STEPS (pedometer measurement)	N SIZE	PAIN CONTROLLED	Keep informed about test and treatment	Adequacy of info to family and friends	Informed about delay	Understanding and caring about patient	OVERALL RATING OF CARE	OVERALL PERCENTILE
BASELINE													
GOAL													
Month/Year													
Month/Year													
Month/Year													
Month/Year													
Month/Year													
Month/Year													
Month/Year													
Month/Year													
Month/Year													
Month/Year													
Month/Year													

To download a full-size version of this sample, go to the *Excellence in the Emergency Department* resource page at www.studergroup.com/excellenceintheED.

Train Your Staff

When you train staff on hourly rounding in the ED, ask them what the eight behaviors look like and why they need to do them. Ask them what "PPD" stands for and why it's so important to be successful rounding hourly in the ED. Perhaps most importantly, make your expectations clear.

Role model and practice. Role model for your staff what you want them to do. Remember, because you will be asking staff to "own" hourly rounding and change even more behaviors, it works only if leaders are already rounding on staff and patients.

The point of role modeling is to help staff understand that none of this is new. It's just better. What's not right about checking patients for pain and updating them on their plan of care? Any good ED nurse is already doing these behaviors. With hourly rounding, we are just asking staff to be more prescriptive. By documenting hourly rounds on the log and using the competency assessment, we can find gaps in consistency. More consistency reduces variance of expected clinical outcomes of patients.

All participants in the ED hourly rounding study were formally trained with a competency assessment. After you train your staff, ask them to do a written self-assessment on everything from how they introduce themselves and PPD to how they perform tasks and document their rounding. Then have an evaluator assess them as well. (Note: A comprehensive hourly rounding training DVD is available at www.studergroup.com and contains everything you need to ensure successful hourly rounding in your ED.)

Figure 8.4

Sample Hourly Rounding Competency Checklist

DATE:					
NAME:					
EMERGENCY DEPARTMENT HOURLY ROUNDING COMPETENCY					
EVALUATOR:	SELF ASSESS		EVALUATOR		
	YES	NO	YES	NO	COMMENTS
INTRODUCTIONS					
Knock on door or ask for permission to enter					
Use AIDET to introduce yourself and co-worker					
Manage up your skill or that of your co-worker					
EXPLAIN HOURLY ROUNDING WHEN ROOMED					
Use key words "very good" care					
Explain hourly rounding an rounding schedule - q 1 hour					
UPDATE WHITE BOARDS					
Place name on white board					
Update status of tests/treatments for patient					
Ask patient what "very good" = document on white board					
ADDRESS PPD - PAIN...PLAN OF CARE...DURATION					
Ask patient to rate their pain					
Update patient on plan of care					
Provide approximate waiting time until disposition					
ASSES THE ENVIRONMENT					
Ensure safety (side rails up, call light in reach)					
PERFORM TASKS					
Complete MD ordered treatments, procedures					
Administer ordered medications					
Address personal needs/questions					
CLOSING					
Communicate when you will return					
Is there anything else I can do for you? I have the time					
Document your round on the log					

To download a full-size version of this sample, go to the *Excellence in the Emergency Department* resource page at www.studergroup.com/excellenceintheED.

And finally, once your staff are rounding hourly on patients, leaders should round on patients to hold staff accountable. Just as I discussed back in Chapter 4 on rounding for outcomes, it's critical to round on patients to validate staff behaviors when you roll out new processes like hourly rounding on patients.

Leaders might say:

- "Our goal is to manage your pain effectively. Did your nurse re-assess your pain level after giving your medication?" or:
- "Our goal is to keep you updated on your plan of care. Has staff explained what you're waiting for and what will happen next?"

This type of leader rounding on patients will validate that the prescribed behaviors for hourly rounding are occurring. It also provides opportunity to harvest reward and recognition for staff and physicians and identifies trends for improvement.

Leaders can also use the log as a way to manage up staff (e.g., "I see from the log that the staff have been rounding on you hourly. Have they asked about your pain? Have they told you how long to expect tests to take?").

If a leader notices that four hours are blank in the log, she can take the log to staff to determine if they are rounding, but perhaps not documenting. In the study, those organizations that adhered to the rounding log clearly had better results than those that did not. Ask staff to close their rounding with the words, "I've done my hourly round and am going to document it here on the log." While it's easy to say, it brings a new level of accountability.

And finally, share your findings from reviewing the logs with staff daily so everyone can adjust and respond to the new information.

Hardwire It

Once staff are consistently rounding, use these tips to ensure everyone is 100 percent compliant and rounding in a standardized way for continuous improvement:

- Validate behaviors through information learned from leader rounding on staff, patients, and discharge phone calls;
- Review rounding logs daily to ensure staff compliance with documentation;
- Review results that leaders have harvested at daily stand-up meetings or "huddles";
- Report results monthly to staff, physicians, and senior leaders. Use the Dashboard for Hourly Rounding in the ED at www.studergroup.com/excellenceintheED;
- Use individualized coaching during monthly one-on-one sessions with employees as needed;
- Reward and recognize without restraint!

There's no question that hourly rounding improves patient care. You'll see it for yourself. Your ED will enjoy more positive word of mouth as a result. But you too will enjoy a new reality: one that is safer, quieter, and more efficient. I have had dozens of ED leaders tell me they never thought they would get their staff to make hourly rounds. Yet once they saw the benefits, they got on board quickly and would never consider going back. Once they knew a better way to provide patient care, their values dictated that they do it!

However, timing is everything with hourly rounding. If your staff are still running around looking for a blood pressure cuff because you haven't rounded on them or helped them hear the patient's voice through leader rounding on patients or discharge phone calls, they are not going to want to begin hourly rounding. **You** must engage employees first before you ask **them** to engage.

But in my experience, once they begin hourly rounding, they understand that it's nothing new. Rather, it's a better, more prescriptive way to do what they've always done. Fewer interruptions give staff more control over their time and work. Really, it's a way for them to take back the ED!

The outcomes from hourly rounding are so rewarding. Once a nurse goes into a patient's treatment room during hourly rounds and finds a patient not breathing or climbing over a bed rail, he will be a believer for life. Hourly rounds keep patients safe.

In fact, sometimes you just never know what will make the difference with a patient. Once I was doing validation rounds in the ED and checked in on a patient with dementia who was being evaluated for altered level of consciousness. I said, "One of our goals is to make sure our nurses check on you hourly. Is that happening consistently?"

To my astonishment, this patient had his first lucid moment since he'd been brought to the ED. He said, "Paul's been in here. He asked me about my pain. He updated me on my plan of care and told me what I was waiting on and that he'd be back in about an hour." Although the patient had not been able to absorb much of the communication during his visit, Paul's key words and hourly rounds certainly worked!

Key Learning Points: Hourly Rounding with Individualized Patient Care in the ED

1. The 2006 Studer Alliance for Health Care study on hourly rounding in the ED tested the impact of three types of rounding on patients in 32 Emergency Departments for six weeks: hourly rounding in the reception and treatment areas; 30-minute rounding in the reception and treatment areas; and hourly rounding with individualized patient care in the reception and treatment areas.

2. Results revealed that rounding every hour in the ED reception and treatment areas reduced LWOBS by 23.4 percent, decreased AMA by 22.6 percent; reduced falls by 54.5 percent; reduced call light usage by 34.7 percent; and 39.5 percent fewer families and patients approached the nursing station. Patient satisfaction also increased between 5 and 20 mean points in all areas measured.

3. The study results also show that hourly rounding with individualized patient care—responding to the top priority of the patient—was at least 33 percent more effective than hourly rounding alone across almost all measures. Because the re search was so strong, we absolutely recommend that you implement individualized patient care with hourly rounding. You'll get results more quickly.

4. Hourly rounding in the ED is an advanced tactic. Leader rounding on staff and patients in the ED must be hardwired first. Introducing discharge phone calls prior to hourly rounding is highly recommended.

5. Tracking results, trends, and opportunities is key to show the impact in the above metrics as well as to calculate the positive financial impact obtained by implementing

hourly rounds. Use a 24-hour rounding log daily and a monthly dashboard. Download free templates at www.studergroup.com/excellenceintheED.

6.   Formalized staff training and competency assessment is key to success. Role modeling and role playing as well as setting clear expectations and accountability standards make a big difference.

7.   Feedback is critical. In the hourly rounding study, higher performing EDs had nurse leaders who gave daily feedback to staff on wins, trends, and opportunities. This drove consistent behaviors for long-term results.

CHAPTER 9

Interdepartmental Communication Tools

*"Coming together is a beginning. Keeping together is
progress. Working together is success."*
—Henry Ford

In the ED, strong interdepartmental relationships are crucial,
but too often relationships break down in the face of time pressures.
Managers often complain that they "don't have time" or "nothing
really changes after we meet."

Why does this happen? Often, I find that leaders with these
complaints haven't formalized a feedback process; aren't consistent
about reward and recognition; don't have clear metrics by which to
measure progress; and don't communicate consistently. And yet,
we are so dependent on our internal customers in the ED!

Everyone *wants* to work well together…to create a great place
for employees to work, physicians to practice, and patients to receive care. But the best intentions can go unnoticed when barriers
get in the way. However, when you use a disciplined process to set
goals, communicate, and follow up, you move ideas to execution
and get results.

Four tools that we will discuss in this chapter are highly effective in building strong interdepartmental relationships and addressing the above barriers: 1) stakeholder meetings; 2) internal

customer rounding; 3) stand-up meetings or "huddles"; and 4) thank-you notes. The goal of all of these tactics is real-time information exchange for better solutions.

Hold a Stakeholder Meeting

In a stakeholder meeting, the objective is to set metrics and share results among all stakeholders in the ED. You'll discuss wins, trends, gaps, and opportunities for improvement.

If you've never held a formal ED stakeholder meeting, pull your leaders together and focus on the team's vision for the ED. Consider your vision for the next two to five years. What are your goals to meet the vision? Who will your success depend upon? This will help you determine who should attend the monthly stakeholder meetings.

Typically, these include the ED medical director, assistant medical director, the nursing director/manager, permanent charge nurses, a few key staff physicians, and key ancillary and support leaders. We recommend also including leaders from Registration, Radiology, Environmental Services, and Security. Ask your CEO, CNO, and Vice President of Support Services to attend at least quarterly to support the group on issues like flow, throughput, team-building, role delineation, and service. This will help drive results and accountability.

In a high-performing ED, stakeholder meetings are held monthly with a formal agenda. Studer Group recommends you use an agenda by pillar, which you can download at www.studergroup.com/excellenceintheED. Plan on meetings that last 60 to 90 minutes. The meetings will be longer in the beginning when ancillary and support department leaders are reporting out and you are developing a work plan. As the team matures, meetings should last no more than 60 minutes.

It's not critical that everyone stay for the entire meeting. For instance, you might consider having Lab and Radiology leaders attend just the first 15 minutes to share data and report out on their results. The goal is to identify trends, wins, and opportunities for improvement.

By ensuring that all stakeholders regularly attend, you will create shared ownership. At one ED that I led, a discussion during a stakeholder meeting about flow and keeping patients informed led to an agreement with security to help us make reception area rounds. The result? They became so invested that they took over our visitor protocol, which was immensely helpful to our staff. They gained a new perspective on turnaround times when they saw the 25 people regularly waiting in the ED. As a result, they were more committed to helping us meet our goal to reduce wait times and keep patients and families informed.

When you set goals and follow-up with all stakeholders present, you will also identify your gaps. Your objective is always to match the goal to the result. Typically, you will find that the barrier to moving forward is either the result of a people or a process issue. If it's a people or leadership issue, that will become apparent to the group. If it's a process problem, the meeting provides work time for you and your colleagues to improve the process and increase efficiency together, without falling prey to the "we/they" syndrome.

What kind of processes might need improvement? Many EDs work with Radiology on turning around plain films within 30 minutes of the time the test is done. Through the stakeholder meeting, you can report on this metric monthly, rewarding and recognizing those individuals who show ownership and results. You can also determine what other processes need to be in place.

So in summary, the stakeholder meeting is a monthly guide to ensure that you are tracking results, objectively looking at your measures, and working through process and people issues to meet your performance targets in the ED.

Internal Customer Rounding

I bet you are already thinking: *How do we agree on the follow-up from the stakeholder meeting? Educate our staff? Make sure it's working?*

That's where internal customer rounding comes in. It's one type of rounding for outcomes. The goal is to drive collaboration and results within the department through hardwired meetings between ancillary and support leaders and the ED leader.

The model looks a bit different from rounding within the department (where the ED leader rounds on direct reports in their areas). In this case, the ED leader is an internal customer of ancillary and support departments, but it's still a shared ownership.

At the stakeholder meeting, you'll determine together how often departments will round on the ED leader and who will initiate the meetings. If you are implementing a new process in Radiology, you might meet 15 minutes weekly to determine how the new process is working. The frequency of internal customer rounding is driven by your goals, but should occur at least monthly.

By scheduling a 15-minute rounding appointment with ancillary and support leaders, the ED leader creates opportunity for work time together to solve challenges and ensure behaviors are aligned. While these quick meetings don't replace impromptu phone calls or check-in time with our colleagues, they do provide workspace to solve issues.

For example, if your department is working on AIDET, you will want to ensure ancillary and support departments are also using AIDET so the patient experience is consistent. Gaining commitment from these department leaders to partner in this effort will increase alignment and accountability and improve staff behaviors and end results.

If you need to improve your cleanliness scores in the ED, it's great to do a weekly walk-through together with the Environmental Services (EVS) leader. Perhaps EVS has responsibility for the fact that the floors aren't clean, but maybe the ED leader needs to talk to staff about the overall lack of orderliness when supplies aren't put away properly. It's shared ownership.

It's similar when it comes to meeting registration goals. Many EDs that Studer Group works with have a goal to register patients within seven minutes. Rounding with the registration manager monthly helps the ED leader keep current on what percentage of patients were registered within seven minutes, how many incomplete secondary registrations there were for that month, the amount of cash collected, and understanding how well the team is meeting the agreed upon metrics.

If 10 percent of all patients have an incomplete secondary registration, the ED leader and Registration leaders co-own the results. Perhaps nurses are discharging patients before they are fully registered. By setting up a process where all patients stop at the discharge desk before leaving, Registration will have an opportunity for one final check in case anything is missing from the account.

If registration is taking more than seven minutes, maybe the problem is that patients in triage are getting missed when they are taken directly to a room. By moving from sequential to more parallel processes, nurses can get information to registrars to start the account while the patient is in triage. The goal is to put processes in place to meet the metric that you set for the goal.

Studer Group recommends that the ED leader meet with leaders in Registration, Radiology, Environmental Services, and Security at least once a month. Meet with the volunteer manager, chaplaincy, food, and lab at least once a quarter, unless something is identified during the stakeholder meeting that dictates a more frequent encounter.

Also, location matters. Where you meet is determined by what you will be doing during that round. For instance, whenever I met with the EVS leader, we always started outside the door of the ED and did a complete a walk-through. We walked the route of the patient to see what our patients saw when they entered the ED reception area, as well as what they saw in the treatment area (e.g., hallways, treatment rooms, bathrooms, etc.).

Use an Internal Customer Rounding Log

After rounding, the ancillary or support leader completes the rounding log and sends a note to the ED leader for follow-up in writing to confirm what was decided and when they will next meet. (See sample internal customer rounding log.)

Figure 9.1

Sample: Internal Customer Rounding Log

Name: Trevor Roberts   Department/Unit: EVS

Dept/Person Rounded on: ED-Stacy Stephens   Date/Week of: October 16th

Key Words or Questions to Focus on: AIDET; Privacy

Tip: *Initially explain the commitment to excellent customer service!*

Steps	Comments	
1. What's working well?	Implementing the floor care schedule is going well. EVS supervisors are working closely with the ED charge nurses to identify rooms and common areas they can get into to provide full floor cleaning/waxing.	
2. Is there anyone I should recognize for doing great work?	**Who** Maria	**What/Why** Doing an excellent job using AIDET and key words around privacy. She is consistently writing her name on the white board.
3. What one or two things could we do better?	Emptying trash cans more often in patient rooms to improve perception of cleanliness. Agreements- Stacy will discuss with her staff and ask them to check/empty trash cans after each patient is discharged. Trevor will ask ED housekeepers to empty trash in each patient room every two hours or more frequently when identified by ED staff. Start date- October 23rd.	
4. Progress update from previous rounding	Continue to follow floor care schedule. Goal is to complete all rooms in next 30 days.	
5. Issues to be addressed for follow up/Next time to meet	Follow up on trash collection. Meet again in two weeks.	

Review findings with your next level leader regularly.

To download a full-size blank version of this template, go to the *Excellence in the Emergency Department* resource page at www.studergroup.com/excellenceintheED.

These tools flow together. At the monthly stakeholder meeting, we identify areas for improvement and processes to work on. As we begin to work on these items, internal customer rounding validates that those things are happening and creates shared ownership between the leaders to move the processes forward. It's important to report back progress at the stakeholder meeting to close the loop.

Stand-Up Meetings or "Huddles"

The goal of stand-up meetings or huddles is real-time knowledge exchange to ensure staff have a successful shift. It offers a quick opportunity to introduce a new employee in the department, reinforce a new clinical protocol, or communicate wins identified through rounding. If you just implemented a new tool—say, bedside report or hourly rounds—you can remind staff about expected behaviors and answer any questions.

Huddles are one of the most effective ways to get information down to the very local level so your staff know what is happening in the department each day. Think of them as a football huddle where the plays are shared and the players are given their roles and responsibilities. You'll communicate both within the department and across departments in the ED at the stand-up meeting.

It works like this: At the beginning of every shift change, gather together all staff for a quick 3 to 5 minute meeting. The charge nurse or clinical leader usually runs the meeting with a standard agenda designed to inform and motivate staff, as well as remind them about expected behaviors that are being hardwired. Begin by talking about what's working well and then reinforce behaviors you're working on.

Run the board so everyone can see who's ready to be discharged and how many patients are in triage and the reception area. The charge nurse can update the group on the status of patients the ED is holding for admission and on anything concerning ancillary or support departments that might affect performance in the ED (e.g., CT scanner down for two hours; housekeeper called in sick). This allows staff to communicate appropriately with patients.

A stand-up meeting agenda might include:

- Quick wins from rounding or a connect-to-purpose letter/ story;
- Review results of goals (e.g., current patient satisfaction scores, LWOBS rate, percent of patients quick registered);
- Review behavior that is being hardwired (e.g., AIDET, hourly rounding);
- Introduction of new staff, if applicable;
- Other brief information that the staff need to give safe care and have a great shift.

Sacred Heart Hospital in Pensacola, FL, is using stand-up meetings to ensure more accurate documentation compliance to improve reimbursement for the ED. Each week, the clinical decision unit nurse and ED leadership incorporate both wins and barriers into the stand-up meeting and recognize staff doing an outstanding job with these efforts.

"The staff work so hard to take care of patients," says Joana Adams, Sacred Heart's Vice President of Operational Projects. "This ensures that their efforts generate quality reimbursement as well. Due to the volume of visits we have, one missing code over a period of a year can result in millions of dollars of missing revenue."

Looking for connect-to-purpose stories to share at stand-up meetings? Harvest them when rounding on staff when you ask, "Who can I recognize for great work?"

Imagine how the team at Upson Regional Medical Center in Thomaston, Georgia, felt when CEO David Castleberry shared this letter with them:

I want to lift up the actions of my coworker Candace Gooden, EMT-I, soon to be RN. She took the extra step to care for a patient, and it shows her professionalism. But most of all, it shows her empathy and compassion.

Our EMS unit was dispatched to a local nursing home to transport a patient with a terminal illness to her residence. Hospice had arranged the move from the skilled nursing facility to her home so she could spend the last few days with family in the dignity of her home. Candace was the tech on this call, getting into the back of the ambulance for the ride to her residence.

As we got underway, Candace asked me to drive slowly and take my time getting to our destination. I wondered to myself, *Why is she asking me to do this?* I could hear Candace talking to the patient, even though she was unable to respond.

After a few minutes, Candace asked me if I had some Chapstick, which she knew I did, and could she borrow it. I gave her my new stick, still sealed. I found out later that during the ride home, Candace had taken a tongue depressor, wrapped it with 4x4s, soaked them with a normal saline flush, and cleaned dried food and medications from the patient's tongue. She then brushed the patient's teeth with more 4x4s and combed her hair. Using a Q-tip, she applied Chapstick to the patient's dried, cracked lips, all the while conversing with this non-verbal woman.

We arrived at our destination, took her inside and placed her into her bed. Before leaving, Candace spoke with a family member, and then returned to speak to our patient one last time, and this time, it sounded as if she responded to Candace.

In the truck, returning to headquarters, I asked Candace why she needed my Chapstick. Candace proceeded to tell me what all she had done for this terminally ill patient on the way home to die. This was not your ordinary patient care. I asked Candace why she did it, and her reply was simply this—the patient's husband was going to be there waiting for his wife to come home, and Candace wanted to ensure that this patient, not long for this world, would look her best, so he would remember his beautiful wife this way.

Special. Extraordinary. Empathetic. Compassionate. That's what Candace is all about. I still get chills down my spine and teary-eyed when I think of the care my partner provided.

Kenny Allen, EMT-Paramedic

How Often to Huddle

The best practice at high-performing EDs that Studer Group coaches is every four hours: at 7 a.m., 11 a.m., 3 p.m., 7 p.m., 11 p.m. and 3 a.m. However, be sure you huddle at least at shift change and keep them short. Some organizations literally use an egg timer to keep them to less than five minutes.

At certain times of day—like at 3 p.m. when the ED is typically busy—we recommend the house supervisor, radiology manager or lead tech, EVS manager, and lab manager attend so everyone is current on turnaround times, ancillary and support issues, and bed status. We also suggest that the ED physician attend while the charge nurse does a quick run of the board.

Who needs a 3 a.m. huddle? you may be asking. At one ED I know, their 3 a.m. huddle became highly effective. If there weren't many patients in the department, they might take that time to do a quick case review of a challenging patient they'd had that day. They had a number of recent nursing graduates then, who were very appreciative of physician education around different cases.

Otherwise, the group might take those few minutes to go clean up the trauma room or an ortho cart. The goal is to keep the huddles consistent around the clock. No opting out!

Huddles don't have to be perfect, so just begin! Also, be sure to control the content to keep them positive and focused. One charge nurse I know told me that her staff complained that huddles had gotten so "negative." Upon reflecting, she realized that they had had so many positive stories, that the group had gradually drifted away from sharing those and would instead get stuck on discussing the far fewer negative patient letters. They needed to get back to the positive.

What's in it for staff? The whole point of this brief meeting at shift change is to exchange quick information…which is why we include physicians, ancillary staff, and support leaders when possible. Huddles also benefit patients because we are more efficient by actively managing flow and throughput. And leaders like the way huddles drive ownership and accountability.

When I was an ED director, I noticed that there were frequently a few nurses who could never seem to make it to any of our daily huddles. Of course, some nurses might be with a sick patient or otherwise busy and may not make it to all huddles, but they should always be able to make it to some. But typically, they were the same nurses who were costing me overtime because they could not complete their work on time by the end of the shift. The nurse who can't make it to the huddles may be the same one who has other performance issues.

Huddles help us learn who we need to spend more time coaching to drive service and efficiency as well as to improve flow and throughput in the department.

Use a Reminder Card

Some EDs will distribute a brief card at the huddle with a reminder of what the group is focusing on. Sacred Heart, for example, used the card below to remind staff about bedside report; report out on patient satisfaction scores on "kept informed"; and to share results from a chart audit on the use of pain protocols.

You might use a card like this for a whole quarter or longer, depending on how long it's taking to hardwire a behavior.

Figure 9.2

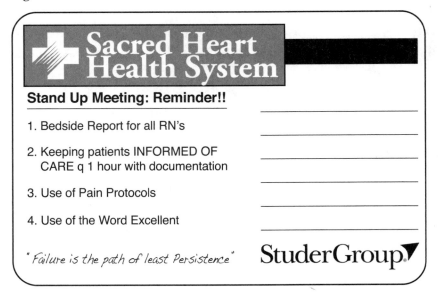

To download a full-size version of this sample, go to the *Excellence in the Emergency Department* resource page at www.studergroup.com/excellenceintheED.

Sample Dialogue from the Charge Nurse at a Stand-Up Meeting

"Good morning! As you can see, our patient satisfaction scores are posted and we are in the 80th percentile this month and we are trending in the 90th percentile for the week. Great work! Our priority is to keep patients informed, so please be sure to check on your patients each hour and inform them about what is going on with their care. Use the word 'informed' because this helps our patients recognize how hard we are trying to provide an explanation. Remember to document 'patient informed regarding care' as was discussed in the unit meeting last week.

"Congratulations to Julie who got a great thank-you note from a patient this week, thanking her for explaining every step of the care provided when her husband came in with a pneumothorax. (Read note.) Letting patients know what to expect and how long it takes clearly makes a difference.

"Welcome to Brad, our new agency RN. Faye is going to be his buddy today, but everyone be sure to help him on the unit today. Thanks for all you do. Let's have a great day."

Huddles are your mainstay of daily communication with staff in the department. Information shared also leads to reward and recognition that can be communicated in a formal thank-you note.

The Power of a Thank-You Note

What gets recognized gets repeated. That's why Studer Group considers personalized Thank-You Notes a "Must Have®." They are one of the very best ways to validate an employee is doing worthwhile work and making a difference.

In the ED, thank-you notes also manage up others to strengthen bonds between coworkers interdepartmentally. **However, you must hardwire leader rounding on staff and patients first so you can harvest these wins.** Rounding will drive your ability to manage up with a thank-you note.

When you round as a leader on staff in the ED, say, for example, "Is there someone you want to recognize? Anyone in Registration who's been really helpful this month as we implemented bedside registration?"

When you learn that Jeanne has been consistent in completing her registrations at bedside, you have a great opportunity to send her a handwritten thank-you note and mail it to her home address.

A caution however: Always check in with the leader of the ancillary or support department before you send a thank-you note to one of his or her employees. Here's why: Let's say I'm rounding and one of my staff tells me that Tina in Radiology did a great job fitting in an urgent patient and getting them quickly to and from the department. What if I send Tina a thank-you note but she happens to be under disciplinary action? Maybe she's hustling because she has to!

So before I send her a thank-you note, I'd just send a quick email to her supervisor: "Hi, Tom. I just learned that Tina did a great job fitting in an urgent patient for us today. If it's appropriate, I'd like to write her a note. Any concerns?"

If Tina is under disciplinary action, her leader may just tell me, "Thanks for letting me know. I will pass on some verbal recognition to Tina, but please hold off on the thank-you note for now."

If everything is okay, her leader is no doubt happy to hear good news from the ED about one of his employees and would encourage me to write the note!

Tips:

Be timely. Time moves fast in the ED, so write thank-you notes the same week you hear about the good deed. When I was a nurse leader, I scheduled time every Friday to write thank-you notes. I also brought blank thank-you notes to charge nurse meetings so we could write them to other departments when we were together.

Be specific. Write: "Rich, I was rounding with Terry and she was so appreciative of the way you are making patients feel comfortable as we're implementing bedside registration. Thank you for helping us reach our goal of registering 100 percent of all eligible patients at the bedside."

Tie it back to your organization's standards of behavior. When John works an extra shift in Radiology, write: "Thank you, John, for working last night. I know you had to sacrifice some family time to be there for us. You really exhibited our Standard of the Month: Commitment to Coworker."

So what's worthy of a thank-you note?

I do a "gut check" when I drop a thank-you note in the mail. I ask myself: *Was this something above and beyond the individual's normal job responsibilities? Has it positively impacted employee, patient, or physician engagement in the ED?*

If yes, I know it was right to send the note. So I use this approach, rather than any type of quota when determining how many to send.

In summary, these four tools are the ones you need to be successful with interdepartmental communication. The stakeholder meeting is a high-level strategic meeting that will keep you on course and determine how well you are meeting the goals you set out for the ED. Internal customer rounding validates that the things you put into place are working and ensures that you do so in partnership with your ancillary and support leaders, so you move together.

Stand-up meetings or huddles are the mechanism for daily communication that your staff need to ensure they do the behaviors every day. They provide opportunity for knowledge exchange, reinforce expected behavior, and reset expectations for local ownership.

As you harvest opportunities to reward and recognize through stakeholder meetings, stand-up meetings, and internal customer rounding, thank-you notes close the loop. The more frequently you reward and recognize, the more likely it is that your employees will repeat the behavior on a daily basis.

Thank-You Notes Turn the Flywheel

They are so powerful. When Greg Pivirotto, CEO of University Medical Center in Tucson, Arizona, rounded on Marsha Peters, he learned that there were plenty of reasons to send a thank-you note to one of Marsha's direct reports, Suzanne Cohen, RN. Read on to see how Greg's detailed thank-you note re-recruits Suzanne...and how Suzanne pays it forward to Marsha. Watch how the flywheel turns!

January 26, 2009

Dear Suzanne,

Recently, while rounding with Marsha Peters, she was singing your praises as one of the department's more experienced nurses and that you are an excellent resource to new staff. She said that you precept and mentor them, with one of them commenting that you are the best nurse she had ever had as a preceptor.

Marsha also told me that you do a really nice job with your patients and are proactive if they have problems or issues, letting her know to follow through so she can help to smooth out concerns or questions. She also stated that you take time to manage up other staff, not just in the department, but for nurses on other floors also. You are very conscientious and come in every day with a smile, willingness to help, and a positive attitude. Marsha also noted that on top of all your regular duties, you also share your knowledge and expertise by helping to teach classes for the department training program.

Suzanne, it is people such as you who make UMC the number one hospital in Arizona, and I thank you for all that you do.

Sincerely,

Gregory A. Pivirotto
CEO

Suzanne writes back:

Dear Greg,

I just came back from getting my mail and much to my surprise and delight, I received a note of appreciation from you. You could knock me over with a feather!

You have no idea—or perhaps you do—how much it means to a nurse, closer in age to 60 than 50, who goes home tired and sometimes wonders why on earth she chose nursing as a profession, to receive a note of appreciation and encouragement from the guy at the top! Thank you so much for taking the time to write and send this...I will treasure it.

By the way, you have a real gem in Marsha Peters... She is the person who keeps us going. I have never met a person in a management position more genuinely concerned about her staff, patients, and always making sure each and every staff member feels valued and appreciated.

Suzanne Cohen, RN

Often it all comes down to gratitude...for what we do, for what others do for us, and for what we can give back. By taking the time to say or write a word of thanks, we not only help others feel good about what they do, we feel better about what we do. So write a thank-you note to someone who went above and beyond. I promise it will make their day!

Key Learnings: Interdepartmental Communication Tools

1. There are four tools that are highly effective in building strong interdepartmental relationships and addressing barriers: 1) stakeholder meetings; 2) internal customer rounding; 3) stand-up meetings or "huddles"; and 4) thank-you notes.

2. Stakeholder meetings are used to set metrics and share results among all stakeholders in the ED. These monthly meetings guide the work plan and typically include the ED medical director, assistant medical director, the nursing director/ manager, permanent charge nurses, a few key staff physicians, and key ancillary and support leaders.

3. Internal customer rounding is one type of rounding for out comes. Ancillary and support leaders round on the ED leader to identify wins, solve challenges, align behaviors, and improve results identified in the stakeholder meeting. There is shared ownership. The ancillary or support leader completes a rounding log to track and follow-up on action items, and progress is reported at the stakeholder meeting.

4. Stand-up meetings or "huddles" gather all staff together for a quick three to five minute meeting at shift change for real-time information exchange that will impact the success of the shift (e.g., new staff, clinical protocols, review of behaviors being worked on).

5. Reward and recognition that is harvested from stakeholder meetings, internal customer rounding, and stand-up meetings can be acknowledged through formal thank-you notes from leaders. For greatest impact, thank-you notes should be specific, handwritten, and mailed to the employee's home.

No ED Left Behind

"There will come a day when you can no longer do this. Today is not that day."
— Franklin Delano Roosevelt

My hope is that after reading this book, you can see that achieving excellence in the Emergency Department is not only attainable but is mission-critical to the long-term survival and success of emergency medicine today and in the future.

Even in the face of multiple challenges like overcrowding, staffing shortages, growing volumes, sicker patients, limited space, aging equipment, ever-changing regulatory requirements, and healthcare reform, many of us have worked our entire careers remaining committed to improving emergency care for our patients and their families.

The reality: ED visits have increased by almost 32 percent between 1996 and 2006, with 119 million visits in 2006 alone. That's equal to one in every five Americans making a visit to an Emergency Department. And it's only going to get worse.[1]

The good news is, we do have the answers to the challenges we face. It starts and ends with leadership. Just as we have placed into law the No Child Left Behind Act, we need to make the same commitment to ensure that there is No ED Left Behind.

By implementing the evidence-based leadership tools and tactics outlined in this book, we can ensure that each patient receives timely, high-quality emergency care...that ED staff feel they have purpose and make a difference every day in the lives of their patients...and that ED physicians feel empowered to make the necessary critical decisions to save lives. That's really what it comes down to: saving lives, restoring health, and creating hope.

Tomorrow is another opportunity to do just that. Your next ED shift might bring you a small child in severe respiratory distress; a violent psych patient hearing voices and threatening harm to you and others; a young father with a wife and three children who dies from an acute myocardial infection after your team performs CPR and ACLS protocols for over an hour; and a beloved grandmother complaining of shortness of breath whose chest X-ray reveals metastatic lung cancer.

The same shift may bring a mom who is grateful that you immediately took her wheezing child back to get help; parents who thank you for your compassion in dealing with their mentally ill daughter; a tearful wife and mother who looks to you for explanation and help in understanding the untimely death of her husband and her young children's father; and a grief-stricken husband who is in imminent danger of losing his beloved wife of 60 years.

In emergency medicine, what we do is never a job. It's a calling.

Every ED has the opportunity to provide excellent care to every patient, every time, with every encounter. Does it require change? Absolutely!

But we're good at change. We deal with it every day. Change is about choice, and choice is about us...and ultimately, it's up to us.

Thank you for your leadership and commitment to saving lives in the Emergency Department. Who knows? The tools you implement today may save your own life—or that of one you love—tomorrow. Let's heed the call.

No ED Left Behind.

Bibliography

Chapter 1

[1] Schuler, A.J. "Overcoming Resistance to Change: Top Ten Reasons for Change Resistance." *Schuler Solutions, Inc.* 2003. <www.schulersolutions.com> (3 July, 2009).

[2] Fleming, Douglas S., and Ann Kilcher. "Organizing and Managing School Change." Workshop held 8 November, 1991. The National Center for Innovation National Conference. Colorado Springs, CO.

[3] Glasscock, Sue, and Kimberly Gram. "Winning Ways: Establishing an Effective Workplace Recognition System." *National Productivity Review* 14, no. 3 (2001): 91-102.

[4] Senge, Peter. *The Fifth Discipline: The Art & Practice of the Learning Organization.* New York: Doubleday, 2006.

Chapter 2

[1] Committee on the Future of Emergency Care in the United States Health System and Board on Health Care Services, Institute of Medicine of the National Academies. *Hospital-Based Emergency Care: At the Breaking Point.* Washington, D.C: The National Academies Press, 2006.

2   "Estimates of Emergency Department Capacity: United States 2007." *Centers for Disease Control and Prevention.* 2007. <www.cdc. gov/nchs/products/pubs/pubd/...capacity/ED_capacity.pdf> (26 June, 2009).

3   Ibid.

4   "RN Supply and Demand Projections." *U.S. Department of Health and Human Services: Health Resources and Services Administration, Bureau of Health Professions.*

5   "Emergency Department Pulse Report." South Bend, IN: Press Ganey Associates, Inc., 2008.

6   Ibid.

7   Murphy, Bob. "Evidence-Based Leadership^{SM} for Reduced Risk." *Managing Infection Control,* July 2007, 64-72.

Chapter 4

1   Studer, Quint. *Hardwiring Excellence.* Gulf Breeze, FL: Fire Starter Publishing, 2003.

2   Ibid.

3   Buckingham, Marcus, and Curt Coffman. *First, Break All the Rules: What the World's Greatest Managers Do Differently.* New York: Simon & Schuster, 1999.

4   Gilboy, Nicki, and Paula Tanabe. "Who Is Leaving the Emergency Department Without Being Seen?" *Advanced Emergency Nursing Journal* 30, no.1 (2008): 3-10.

Chapter 5

[1] Forster, A., et al. "The Incidence and Severity of Adverse Events Affecting Patients After Discharge from the Hospital." *Annals of Internal Medicine* 138, no. 3 (2003): 161-74.

[2] "Adverse Drug Events Occurring Following Hospital Discharge." *Journal of General Internal Medicine* 20, no. 4 (2005): 317-23.

[3] Clark, P.A. *Patient Satisfaction and the Discharge Process: Evidence-Based Best Practices.* Marblehead, MA: HCPro, Inc., 2006.

[4] Forster, A., et al. "The Incidence and Severity of Adverse Events Affecting Patients After Discharge from the Hospital." *Annals of Internal Medicine* 138, no. 3 (2003): 161-74.

[5] Ibid.

Chapter 6

[1] Institute of Medicine (IOM). *To Err is Human: Building a Safer Health System.* Washington, DC: National Academies Press, 2004.

[2] Ibid.

[3] Kizer, K.W. "Patient Safety: A Call to Action: A Consensus Statement from the National Quality Forum." *Medscape General Medicine.* 2001. <http://www.medscape.com/mgmhome?src-hdr> (28 December, 2004): 1-11.

[4] "National Patient Safety Goals." Oakbrook Terrace, IL: Joint Commission, 2009.

5 Runy, Lee Ann. "Patient Handoffs." *H&HN Magazine*, May 2008, 40-47.

Chapter 7

1 Makoul, G., A. Zick, and M. Green. "An Evidence-Based Perspective on Greetings in Medical Encounters." *Archives of Internal Medicine* 167, no. 11 (2007): 1172-6.

2 Ibid.

3 "Pulse Report 2009 Emergency Department: Patient Perspectives on American Health Care." South Bend, IN: Press Ganey Associates, Inc., 2009.

4 Keating, N.L., et al. "Patient Characteristics and Experiences Associated With Trust in Specialist Physicians." *Annals of Internal Medicine* 164 (2004): 1016-2l.

5 "Factors Affecting Drug Response." In *Merck Manual of Diagnosis and Therapy*, edited by M.H. Beers and R. Berkow, 2574-87. Whitehouse Station, NJ: Merck Research Laboratory, 1999.

Chapter 8

1 Meade, Christine M., Amy L. Bursell, and Lyn Ketelsen. "Effects of Nursing Rounds on Patients' Call Light Use, Satisfaction, and Safety." *American Journal of Nursing* 106, no. 9 (2006): 58-70.

2 "Emergency Department Rounding Study." *Studer Alliance for Health Care Research*. Gulf Breeze, FL: Studer Group, 2007.

Resources

Accelerate the momentum of your Healthcare Flywheel^{SM}.
Access additional resources at www.studergroup.com/excellenceintheED.

Magazines:

Hardwiring Results: Excellence in the Emergency Room, Issue 5, 2006
This issue focuses on excellence in the Emergency Department. Article topics include boosting ED reimbursement, improving patient safety with ED communication tools, reducing patients who leave without treatment, and more.

Hardwiring Results: Return on Investment, Issue 8, 2007
This issue focuses on return on investment with article topics such as calculating ROI in the Emergency Department and finding new revenue in your Emergency Department, and provides a link to an ED calculator.

Visit www.studergroup.com to view additional *Hardwiring Results* magazines.

Books:

Hardwiring Excellence
Quint Studer helps healthcare professionals to rekindle the flame

and offers a road map to creating and sustaining a Culture of Service and Operational Excellence that drives bottom-line results.

Eat THAT Cookie! How Workplace Positivity Pays Off...For Individuals, Teams and Organizations
Written by Liz Jazwiec, RN, is packed with realistic, down-to-earth tactics leaders can use right now to infuse positivity into their culture.

Engaging Physicians: A Manual to Physician Partnership
A new book by Dr. Stephen C. Beeson, is a tested, staged approach to create physician loyalty, improve physician partnership, and generate superior organizational performance.

Hardwiring Flow: Systems and Processes for Seamless Patient Care
By Drs. Thom Mayer and Kirk Jensen, dives into one of the most critical issues facing healthcare leaders today: patient flow. After reading this book, you will learn how patient flow helps organizations maximize the "Three Es": *Efficiency, Effectiveness,* and *Execution.*

For more information about these books or to view additional books, visit www.firestarterpublishing.com.

Webinar Tracks:

Engaging Physicians
Presented by Stephen Beeson, MD

Dealing with "Special" Colleagues: Discouraging Disruptive Behavior
Presented by Gerald Hickson, MD, Faculty, Vanderbilt University Medical Center

<u>Physician Accountability: Aligning Physician Performance with Organizational Goals to Drive Clinical and Financial Outcomes</u>
Presented by Wolf Schynoll, MD, FACEP

For more information on Studer Group's webinar tracks, visit www.studergroup.com/webinars.

DVD Training Resources:

<u>Emergency Department Rounding</u>
This DVD provides the how-to's for implementing Emergency Department hourly rounding on patients to improve safety, quality, and patient satisfaction, and shows what hourly rounding looks like with use of vignettes shot in a large emergency room.

<u>AIDET^{SM} Five Fundamentals of Patient Communication</u>
AIDET—Acknowledge, Introduce, Duration, Explanation, and Thank You—is a powerful communication tool. When interacting with patients, gaining trust is essential for obtaining patient compliance and improving clinical outcomes. AIDET is a simple acronym that represents how we can gain trust and communicate with people who are nervous, anxious, and feeling vulnerable. Studer Group has created AIDET as a comprehensive training tool that will enhance communication within your organization.

<u>Building Patient Trust with AIDET Training DVD</u>
The Building Patient Trust with AIDET training DVD is ideal for training staff, leaders, and physician groups on how to use the key communication steps of AIDET: Acknowledge, Introduce, Duration, Explanation and Thank You. Participants will learn the what, why, and how of reducing patient anxiety, improving clinical outcomes, and creating a better patient experience with AIDET.

HighMiddleLow™ Performer Conversations
It is crucial that any organization have a method to re-recruit high performers, continue to develop middle performers, and move low performers "up or out" of the organization. If not, organizations hit a wall where progress slows and they cannot achieve their full potential. Based on work with hundreds of healthcare organizations, Studer Group has developed a critical management approach for moving organizational performance called highmiddlelow.

For more information on Studer Group solutions or DVD training resources, visit www.firestarterpublishing.com.

Institutes:

Nuts and Bolts of Operational Excellence in the Emergency Department
Improve patient flow and build service and operational excellence in your Emergency Department as Jay Kaplan, MD, FACEP, and Stephanie Baker, RN, MBA, CEN, both with extensive and ongoing real-life ED experience, share proven tactics such as Provider in Triage, Rounding for Outcomes, Discharge Phone Calls, Key Words at Key Times, and AIDET.

Practicing Excellence: The Physician Institute
Studer Group has designed a staged approach to engaging physicians to achieve clinical, service, and operational excellence. Studer Group physician coach experts provide participants evidence-based tactics to take back home to achieve and sustain measurable results in patient satisfaction, physician satisfaction, employee retention, and clinical outcomes. After leaving this institute, healthcare leaders will know the answer to the question, "How do we get physicians on board?"

Taking You and Your Organization to the Next Level with Quint
Studer

Learn the tools, tactics, and strategies that are needed to Take You
and Your Organization to the Next Level at this two-day institute
with Quint Studer and Studer Group's coach experts. You will walk
away with your passion ignited, and with Evidence-Based Leadership[SM] strategies to create a sustainable culture of excellence.

What's Right in Health Care[SM]

One of the largest healthcare peer-to-peer learning conferences in
the nation, *What's Right in Health Care* brings organizations together
to share ideas that have been proven to make healthcare better.

To review a listing of Studer Group institutes or to register for an
institute, visit www.studergroup.com/institutes.

For information on continuing education credits, visit www.studer-group.com/cmecredits.

Coaching:

Emergency Department Coaching

Is a comprehensive approach to improving service and operational
efficiency in the Emergency Department. Our team of ED coach
experts will partner with you to implement best practices, proven
tools, and tactics using our Evidence-Based Leadership approach to
improve results in all five pillars: People, Service, Quality, Finance,
and Growth. Key deliverables include decreasing staff turnover,
improving employee, physician, and patient satisfaction, decreasing door to doctor times, reducing left without being seen rates,
increasing upfront cash collections, and increasing patient volumes
and revenue.

To learn more about Studer Group coaching, visit www.studer-group.com.

About Studer Group:

Studer Group's mission is to change the face of healthcare by creating a better place for employees to work, physicians to practice medicine, and patients to receive care. Studer Group is an outcomes-based healthcare performance improvement firm that coaches hundreds of hospitals, health systems, medical practices, and end-of-life organizations to achieve and sustain clinical results. To learn more about Studer Group, visit www.studergroup.com.

Visit www.studergroup.com/excellenceintheED to access and download many of the resources, examples, and tools mentioned in *Excellence in the Emergency Department*.

Acknowledgments

I would like to thank:

Quint Studer for your endless passion to improve healthcare, your uncanny ability to inspire others, and your willingness to continuously coach all of us to deliver better results for every patient, every time. Thank you for being our fearless leader!

BG Porter for your support of the ED work, taking time to read the very first rough draft of this book, and for being a role model to all of us at Studer Group of what an executive leader should and can be.

Barbara Hotko for encouraging me to write this book even before I had an outline and for your unconditional love, relentless mentorship, and sheer tenacity to always push me to give my best in every situation. Hottie, I adore you and am grateful for each moment I have with you!

Lynne Cunningham for your friendship, mentoring me (especially in the early years when I was as green as grass!), and for reading the manuscript and offering recommendations that greatly improved the end product. Lynne, you mean the world to me!

Stacy Tompkins for keeping me in the right place at the right time all the time. Thank you for your daily encouragement and for always making me laugh. You are an angel!

Chris Román for your tireless efforts editing the manuscript again and again! Your expert knowledge, insight, and guidance made this book what it is today. I appreciate you deeply for helping me realize my dream. Thanks, my friend!

Bekki Kennedy for bringing this book to print and guiding me with skill and confidence each step of the way on my maiden journey.

Jeanne Martin for always offering the right advice at the right time.

Jay Kaplan and Julie Kennedy for your passion for emergency medicine and inspiring me even before I began this journey.

Faye Sullivan, Julie O'Shaugnessy, Terry Rose, and Kat Davis for helping me create the ED coach toolkit. What fun we had!

The entire Studer Group family for your support, friendship, and unwavering commitment to our mission, vision, and values.

My client partners for the opportunity to work with such wonderful and diverse organizations and such passionate and inspired leaders.

Trevor Wright for your friendship and willingness to work with me in the early years when my skills as a leader left much to be desired. Thanks for helping me avoid unnecessary career moves!

MyLil Ramey and Jeannie Wilson for being such great colleagues and friends during our glory years!

Pauline Thomas, Alison McManus, Samantha Meyerhoff, Anthony Ferkich, Paul Manos, and the rest of the original Paradise Valley ED team for your passion to achieve excellence in the face of daily challenges and for never giving up. You guys rock!

Kim and Trevor Roberts for your unconditional friendship and love.

Carol Dunmire for supporting me and keeping me fed (literally!) through my lean years as a new nurse. I still owe you lots of dinners!

My aunt and uncle, Paul and Roberta Pratt, for your lifelong love, encouragement, and support. Thank you for always believing in me.

The Williams and Baker families for your love and prayers and for raising me in a Christian home that always keeps God first and family second.

About the Author

Stephanie Baker is a coach, account leader, and national speaker for Studer Group, perhaps most respected for her ability to consistently deliver superior results through individualized coaching with client partners nationwide.

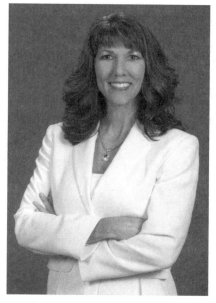

With 20 years of clinical nursing and administrative experience in emergency, trauma, flight, and critical care medicine, she also leads Studer Group's Emergency Services Division and serves as keynote speaker for its two-day "Nuts and Bolts of Service and Operational Excellence in the Emergency Department" Institute. A two-time winner of Studer Group's Pillar Award, Stephanie excels at motivating senior leaders and staff to implement evidence-based tactics that drive accountability and create a culture of "always."

Prior to joining Studer Group in 2005, she was the Director of Emergency Services at Paradise Valley Hospital in San Diego, CA. In her role there, Stephanie moved the Emergency Department from the 4th to the 98th percentile in patient satisfaction, reduced patients who left without treatment from 8 percent to 2.9 percent, and implemented a new "Wipe Out Waiting" bedside registration that contributed to a 20 percent volume increase over 18 months.

Stephanie is a graduate of San Diego State University and holds a bachelor of science degree in nursing and a dual master's degree in business administration and health care management. She was also the recipient of the prestigious "Tribute to Women in Industry" (TWIN) Award in 2004.

With a personal philosophy of "Sometimes we get only one chance," Stephanie's goal is to make a difference with every patient, every time.

How to Order Additional Copies of

Excellence in the Emergency Department
How to Get Results

Orders may be placed:

Online at:
www.firestarterpublishing.com
www.studergroup.com

By phone at: 866-354-3473

By mail at: Fire Starter Publishing
913 Gulf Breeze Parkway, Suite 6
Gulf Breeze, FL 32561

(Bulk discounts are available.)

Excellence in the Emergency Department
is also available online at www.amazon.com.